the vagina book

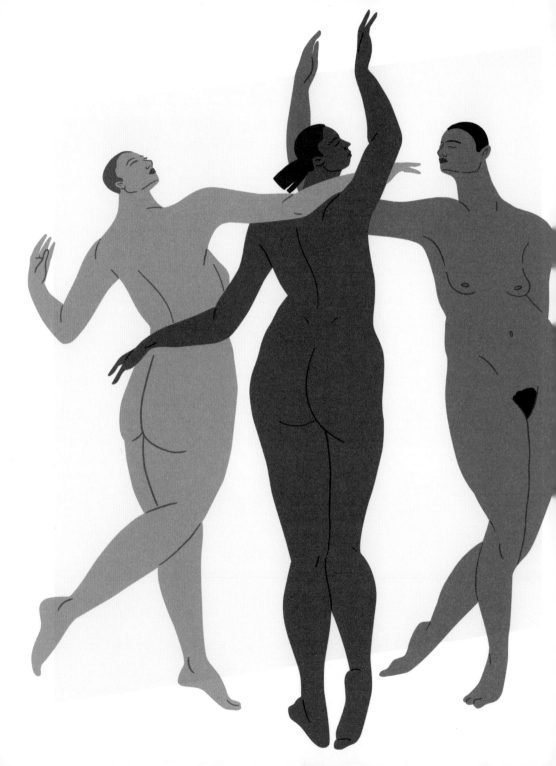

an owner's
manual for
taking care
of your
down there

the
vagina
book

Thinx

with Dr. Jenn Conti, MD

Illustrations by
Daiana Ruiz

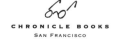

CHRONICLE BOOKS
SAN FRANCISCO

Library of Congress Cataloging-in-Publication Data available.

ISBN 978-1-4521-8244-5

Manufactured in China.

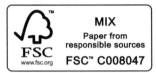

Design by Vanessa Dina.
Illustrations by Daiana Ruiz.

10 9 8 7 6 5 4 3 2

Chronicle books and gifts are available at special quantity discounts to corporations, professional associations, literacy programs, and other organizations. For details and discount information, please contact our premiums department at corporatesales @chroniclebooks.com or at 1-800-759-0190.

Chronicle Books LLC
680 Second Street
San Francisco, CA 94107

www.chroniclebooks.com

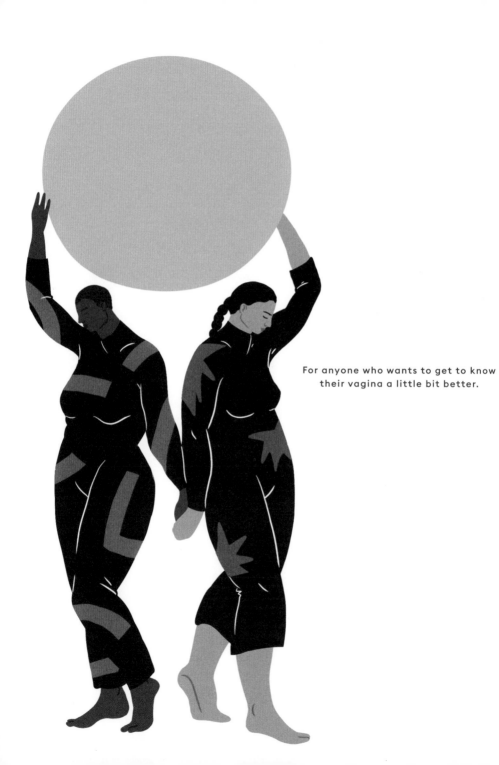

For anyone who wants to get to know
their vagina a little bit better.

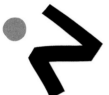

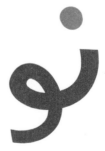

foreword

by Margaret Cho

I don't have my period anymore. It's weird—I miss it.
I never thought I would actually miss it. My monthly
flow was always a hurricane, blowing through me
every 28 days without any thought to what I might
have preferred to be doing. I bled hard throughout my
career highs and lows, falling in love and breaking up,
marriages and divorces, traveling all over the world
and staying home.

My monthly bleed was a constant. I counted on it—like
that annoying friend who shows up, not quite unan-
nounced, but whose visit you conveniently blocked out
because you would so much rather they didn't come.
But then it finally happened: My period broke up
with me and decided never to darken my door (or my
panties, sheets, sofas, dining room chairs, or even
floors) ever again. Now, I surprise myself with my grief.
The mystery of my menses leaving me was, at first, as
baffling as when it originally came.

I didn't have a proper education about my period. I didn't have proper education on anything about my body. My generation was treated to fifth-grade film strips that flickered and stuttered from the classroom projector, while the boys were sent to another classroom to play "Heads Up, 7 Up." These ancient strips of celluloid were meant to let us in on the magic of womanhood, but in truth they were just very long commercials for maxi pads and sanitary belts. That's right, I said *belts*! I am that old. I just had to wing it—in the era before maxi pads had wings! No one told me that the thick black hair that crowded the follicles of my head would now sprout between my legs and under my arms. I had to provide my own answers to why my chest felt sore most of the time, and why many days of the month I would want to cry and scream for seemingly no reason. Puberty was a crazy "choose your own adventure" mystery to which I was provided no clues.

My first period stunned and scared me—that dark blood bubbling out of my crotch was unexpected and startling. I told my mother, who got me a giant box of maxi pads (which felt, most days, like I was riding a brick). She showed me an elaborate method for their disposal.

"You have to roll this up and wrap and wrap and wrap with toilet paper." She demonstrated by winding the toilet paper around the offending used pad until it was a large mass of white paper, roughly the size of a newborn baby. "Then, you cannot throw this in the bathroom garbage can!" she shouted, as she cast an angry glance over at the tiny, plastic trash receptacle next to the toilet. "You have to take it downstairs and put it in the kitchen garbage!" We walked down together to the kitchen so I could watch her as she put the toilet paper/maxi pad baby into a brown paper shopping bag and buried it deep into the kitchen trash, safe underneath the banana peels and coffee grounds. She closed the lid hard and lowered her voice, "Nobody should see it."

Of course, rebel that I am, I would leave the monstrously large and bloodied maxi pads on the back of the toilet, on the floor, or in my white canopy bed. I don't think my pads ever made it into any trash can. I don't hide anything—this is my nature.

My mother never said anything else about it. She knew I was actively disobeying her, but she was also too mortified to stop me. Her silence continued after her hysterectomy, which she never spoke of except to say she was "Finally free . . . feels so good!"

Since most of the women in my family had had the same operation (hysterectomies being absolutely de rigueur in the '70s), I don't have a blueprint of how my people age out of the system—that blood system that "makes a girl a woman." If I had a do-over, I would ask lots of questions and force answers from my silent tribe of women who bury their pads.

Things are totally different today. You're the luckiest bleeders in history. I really mean it. You're living in the Golden Age of Menstruation! I envy you! We live in a time where questions can be answered in the flash of a Google search. (The quality of those answers, however, is another story.) We have products the young girl in me marvels at every day. I can't even imagine what ease a product like Thinx would have given me. Even better, now they've put all the knowledge about the mysteries and secrets we seek in one place. We desperately need resources like this to strip away the lies, misconceptions, and shame around the bodies of over half the world's population! It makes me wish for my period again just so that I could have my questions answered and live my very best, bloody life.

An accomplished performer in all formats, Margaret Cho could be called the "Queen of All Media," having conquered the worlds of film, television, books, music, and theater. She has five Grammy Award nominations (two for music albums, *Cho Dependent* and *American Myth*) and one Emmy nod for her groundbreaking work on *30 Rock*. Never one to shy away from a difficult or "taboo" topic, her socially aware brand of stand-up comedy has made her both a thought leader as well as a teacher to those with open minds and open hearts.

introduction

how I unlearned everything I thought
I believed about vaginas

by Dr. Jenn Conti

I am an ob/gyn doctor: I deliver babies, I do pap smears and breast cancer screenings, I surgically remove uteruses and ovaries, and I perform abortions, because *all* of this is part of healthcare. Inclusivity and choice are guiding principles in my work. But I wasn't always this way. Anyone who knew me as a teenager might not recognize the woman I am today.

When I was sixteen years old, I considered myself to be "pro-life." I thought abortion was murder. I thought anyone who considered it was selfish, coldhearted, and godless. In the community I grew up in, it was common to believe that abortion was the pinnacle of evil in the world. So pervasive was this mentality that "killing babies" was, not infrequently, the topic of social group discussions. If we could just get other people to see how truly black and white the topic of abortion was, they'd surely recognize the moral depravity of the issue, the injustice for the unborn. I wanted to be an ob/gyn doctor because, as the eldest of nineteen grandchildren, I had seen birth, in all its glory, eighteen times over. I wanted to help bring babies into the world, not shut them out of it. I, of all people, *knew* how wrong abortion was.

I started volunteering at a local women's health clinic after school, and it wasn't long before I noticed small, unexpected shifts in my perspective.

One day, a girl I recognized from class came in requesting a whole slew of STI (sexually transmitted infection) tests. She said she'd been at a party the night before and then woke up that morning in a bed she didn't recognize, next to a guy whose name she didn't even know. She said she was pretty sure they'd had sex, and she thought they'd used a condom, but couldn't be sure. Could I just please ask the doctor to order the tests and maybe give her some pills for the next time it happened? Oh, and could I not look at her "like that," like this was the most shocking thing I had ever heard? I remember the feeling of ranking my health decisions against those of other people—that one of them was right and the other was wrong. I never thought of myself as outwardly judging others, but that's exactly what it was: judgment. I assumed I knew what was best for other people, and that scenarios like if, when, and how to parent were one size fits all.

Slowly, stories like this began to lose their sacrilegious bite. Everyone, it appeared, was having sex, and everyone was running into sticky situations like this one.

And instead of getting angry, I got worried. Clearly admonition and religious persuasion were ineffective when it came to sex. What if that was all wrong? What if judgment did more harm than good?

Then the unthinkable happened. Someone I knew, a church leader's daughter, got knocked up, and I knew *she* wasn't godless. If anyone had a direct line to the Almighty, it was "Mary" (because that's the kind of pseudonym you use for a story like this).

Mary was my age and had everything going for her. She had long, gorgeous blond hair that hung beautifully down her back, perfect skin, and a symmetrical smattering of freckles on her cheeks that made you think instantly of midwestern virtue and all things patriotic.

She was dating a boy (let's call him "Ben") and the both of them had attended church every week since they were born. Everyone knew they would probably get married. Ben had given Mary a promise ring—an outward symbol of their love and a public broadcasting of their vow to "keep it in their pants" until their union was approved by Jesus on their wedding night. This was the norm for teenagers in the church.

I still remember the day she came into the clinic. It was late in the afternoon and the facility was about to close. The receptionist called me, saying the last patient had just arrived, 20 minutes late for her appointment, but insisted on being seen, saying it was urgent. She said the girl was hysterical and would need someone to escort her to the exam room. I walked up front, and when I turned the corner into the waiting room, I was dumbstruck. There was church Mary, Ben's Mary, chastity-belt-on-her-ring-finger Mary, and holy-shit-it's-you Mary. Her freckles were obscured by the beet-red shine of her wet, puffy cheeks, but it was unmistakably her.

I took her back to the exam room, and her story came tumbling out. She was pregnant—twelve weeks—and Ben didn't know. Nobody knew (except God, obviously). She worried about what this could mean for her future. She said if she was forced to have a baby, it would ruin her life. There was only one way out of this, and she had already thought about it long and hard. She needed an abortion, and would the clinic please, please, help her? And we did.

When you grow up only seeing one side of an issue, it's easy to *know* the view you hold is the right view. I've spent a lot of time thinking about how I could have so adamantly believed abortion was definitively wrong, and not a complex, often uncomfortable, yet necessary reality of life.

Part of it, I'm sure, came from the fact that I was essentially indoctrinated to think homosexuality, abortion, and interracial marriage were bad. When you teach a child something before the age of seven—the classic developmental cognitive, emotional, and moral stage where we become more capable of rational thought—you're essentially cementing perceived truths into place. And so, this was my truth until I studied science, had some really wonderful teachers, and made friends with people who did not share a similar life story.

Given the 180-degree turn I've made with all of these beliefs, you might think I'd be embarrassed of who I used to be. The truth is, I'm proud of the change I've made because it makes me a better doctor and human to have understood these different assumptions so intimately.

It's this familiarity with a judgmental mindset that has made me the doctor and the educator I am today. At the core of every encounter I have with a patient is the acknowledged truth that no two human beings are alike, and that I will never purport to know what is best for someone else's life. I strive to be an empathetic health provider for those who walk through my clinic door, a teacher, and a resource for anyone who wants to get to know their body a little bit better.

This is exactly what I hope this book will be for others—an honest, compassionate, and inclusive resource. Textbooks and sex ed class can teach us only so much in this area, and vaginal health is certainly not the forte of religious or political leaders. Stories and lived experiences are what round out the most significant narratives, and so, this book is for anyone looking to learn more about vaginas.

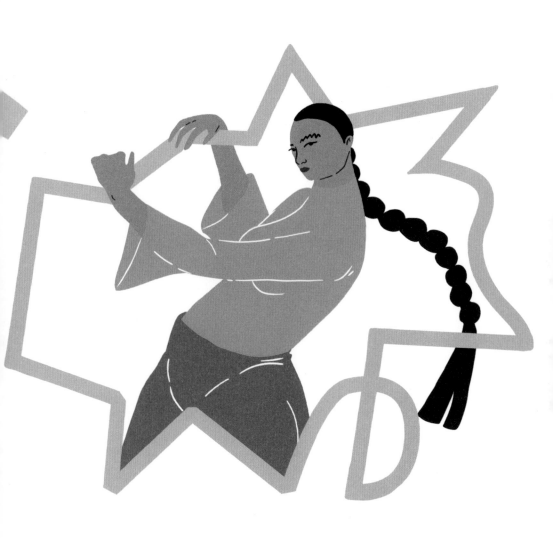

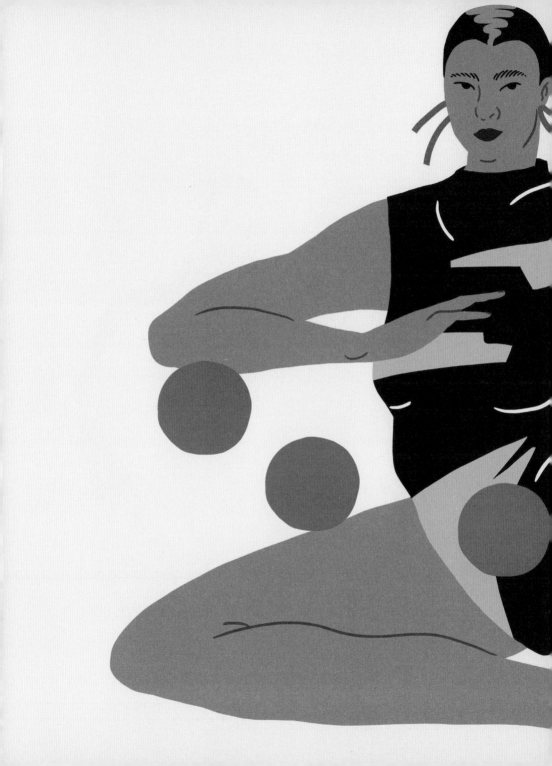

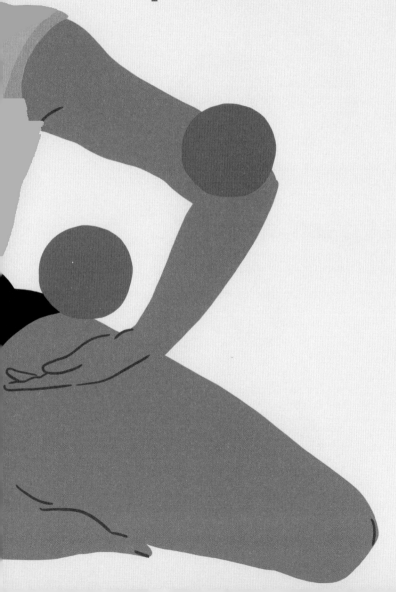

CHAPTER 1

periods

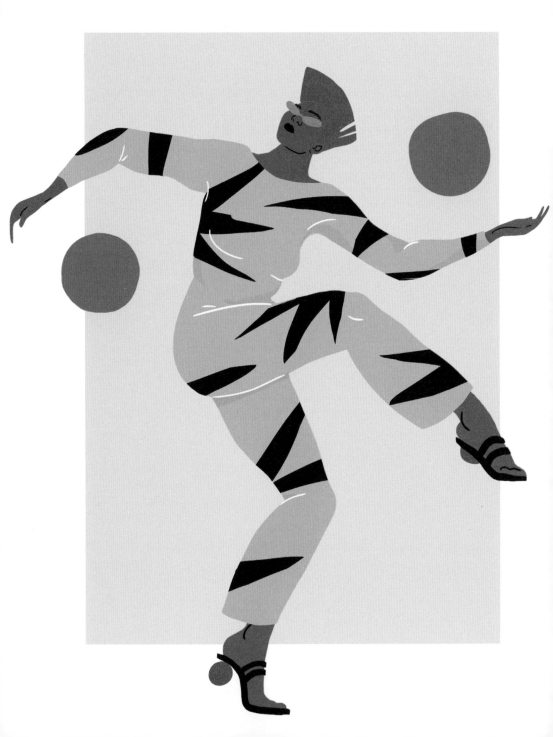

what actually happens during menstruation?

While most of us received a rudimentary education about periods in grade school (which probably involved first kicking all the boys out of the room), it's possible the specifics have become a bit fuzzy since then. Here's the thing—on average, you'll menstruate for over 2,000 days in your lifetime. That's a lot of time to be kind of hazy on the details! So, let's take this opportunity to go back to the basics: What's actually going on down there all month?

In a nutshell, if you menstruate, your body is always preparing for one of its eggs to be fertilized. The lining of your uterus will thicken around one of your eggs, creating a cozy home in preparation for a fertilized egg. If you don't become pregnant, your body sheds the lining and releases the unfertilized egg. Then, the cycle starts all over again! Let's break that down.

menstruation

Day 1 of your period is also day 1 of your whole menstrual cycle. This is when your body gets rid of unneeded stuff: the uterine lining, the unfertilized egg, and mucus. And of course, blood flows out your uterus through your vagina and into your pad, cup, or tampon—or onto your jeans, if you're free bleeding! As you're probably aware, menstruation tends to last 3 to 7 days and is accompanied by all sorts of fun things like cramping, mood swings, fatigue, and more.

follicular phase

Did you know we're born with all the eggs we'll ever have? We usually start with 1 to 2 million follicles (immature eggs), but by the time puberty comes and menstruation begins, the number has dropped to around 400,000. These immature eggs are stored in our ovaries, each inside its own microscopic, fluid-filled follicle. The follicular phase begins when 1 of about 20 competing follicles matures into an egg and ends with ovulation of 1 egg. The first day of your period coincides with your follicular phase, so you're technically double-booked with menstruation for the first week.

Let's talk hormones: In our brains, we have a gland called the hypothalamus, which is responsible for things like thirst, hunger, sleep, sex drive, and hormones. At the beginning of your cycle, the hypothalamus kicks things into gear by telling its buddy, your pituitary gland, to release follicle-stimulating hormone (FSH) and luteinizing hormone (LH). That's when your follicle matures and starts preparing for ovulation, the next phase of menstruation. These multitasking follicles then release another hormone, estrogen, which causes the lining of your uterus to thicken in preparation for the fertilization of your egg.

ovulation

Once your estrogen levels hit their highest point, your hypothalamus gets another message: Release a burst of LH. This surge causes one follicle to burst open and release an egg, which then travels into your fallopian tube. Ovulation typically lasts 1 day, usually around the 14-day mark of your cycle. Tracking when your period starts and ends can give you a better sense of when you ovulate. This is especially useful if you're trying to get pregnant, or if you're not using hormonal birth control and trying to avoid having sex when you're fertile.

If you're using hormonal birth control like the pill, you usually won't ovulate because the constant level of synthetic hormones prevents the peak that kicks off ovulation. The bleeding you may experience every month when you take a pill break is actually not a period at all; it's withdrawal bleeding that's caused by your body taking a break from those hormones.

luteal phase

The luteal phase is when premenstrual syndrome (PMS) kicks in, with mood swings, bloating, fatigue, cravings—you know the drill. The follicle that popped that egg out then transforms into the corpus luteum. The corpus luteum releases progesterone that stabilizes your thickened uterine wall in anticipation of you becoming pregnant. Here's where the road forks: If your egg was fertilized, your body will need its uterine lining to remain thick, so the embryo will begin to produce human chorionic gonadotropin (hCG), the hormone that shows up on a positive pregnancy test. But if your body is sure there's no potential fetus, your estrogen and progesterone levels will decrease, and your uterine lining will begin to disintegrate, which will lead to the beginning of your period.

Now we're back to square one, day 1 of your period, and you get to start the cycle all over again. (Yay!/?) The good news is that the more familiar you get with what's going on with your body, the better you can prepare for each phase.

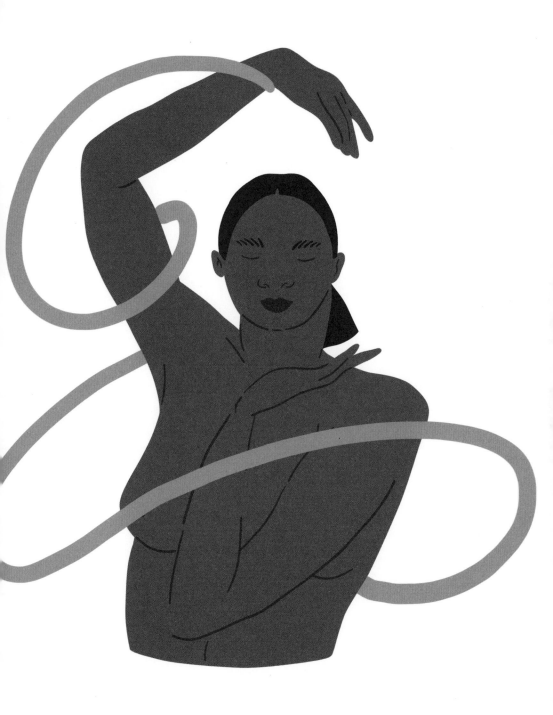

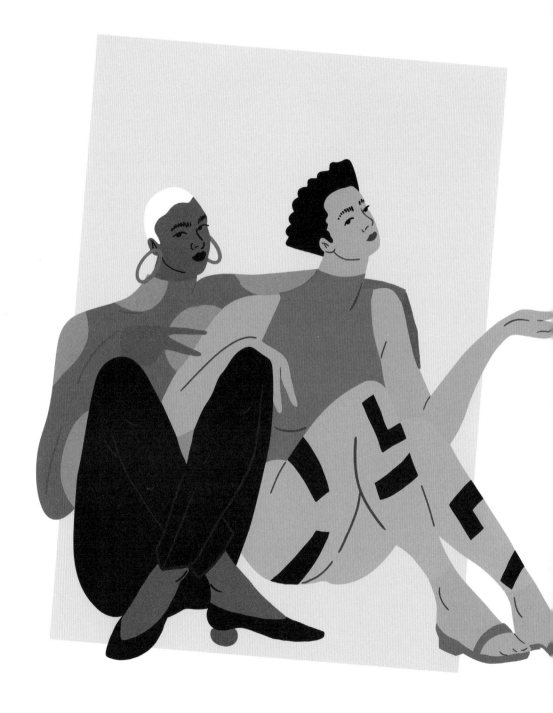

debunking common menstruation myths

Since the dawn of time, people have relied on myths, legends, and whispers to explain what frightens them or what they don't understand. Mankind has a long and frustrating history of misunderstanding bodies with vaginas—especially when it comes to periods. There have been some truly bonkers ideas about menstruation that have been put to rest: Menstruating women can control the weather! Period blood will kill your crops, but it can also cure leprosy! (Need we go on?) Sadly, there are plenty of menstruation myths that have stubbornly persisted, despite evidence to the contrary. Let's talk about a few of the most common (and totally false!) theories.

period blood is dirty blood

It's easy to understand why this one persists. Since many parts of history read as one long "I don't want women to do that" book, using periods as an excuse to tell ladies they are too dirty to do basic things like go to school, make sushi, or have sex is a logical part of that warped agenda. The truth is, while your menstrual flow includes more than just blood, the actual blood that comes out of your vagina is the same as what comes out of a cut, a nosebleed, or anything else.

your cycle should be 28 days

Feeling like your body is different from everyone else's can often turn into feeling like something is wrong with *you*. If your cycle isn't 28 days, that doesn't necessarily mean there's an issue. When people discuss periods, they usually refer to the "average" cycle, which is 28 days, but cycles can actually vary from 21 to 45 days in young teens and 21 to 35 days in adults.

One of the best ways to get to know your flow is by tracking your cycle, whether manually on your calendar or by using an app. Tracking your cycle over time can help you avoid things like mistaking a long cycle for a skipped period. While a shorter, longer, or irregular cycle might be normal for you, it's still a good idea to discuss your cycle with your doctor to rule out any other issues.

people with periods sync up

"But wait!" you might be saying. "I've experienced this—my sister/roommate/coworker and I get our periods at the same time—it can't be a myth!" There's definitely something nice about believing in the magical powers of collective uteruses, but since there's no medical research that suggests the existence of cycle syncing, this probably has a lot more to do with basic math than science. Think about it: A period can last 2 to 7 days, a cycle can last from 21 to 35 days, and these time spans are even wider when you're a teen, so people are bound to bump into each other while they're surfing the crimson wave at some point.

you can't get pregnant during your period

Considering your fertile window is only 5 days long during ovulation, you'd think it would be easy to avoid pregnancy for people who want to do so. Knowing that fact, you'd think you should be in the clear during your period, but remember, the average 28-day cycle doesn't apply to everyone. The number of "safe" days right before or after your period increases with longer cycles and lessens with shorter cycles; if your cycle is shorter, ovulation can occur earlier. And don't forget: Sperm can live inside a vagina for up to 5 days! (Eek!) So, if you and your partner are down for period sex and pregnancy is a possibility you'd like to avoid, don't skip contraception.

your period will attract wild animals

Do you know how many people have been killed by falling coconuts? Enough that it warranted its own Wikipedia page. (Seriously, go check! We'll wait.) By contrast, there has been no evidence to corroborate the very popular idea that if you go swimming during your period, sharks will attack you, or that bears will attack you on the campground. Don't let your flow keep you from getting yo' nature on!

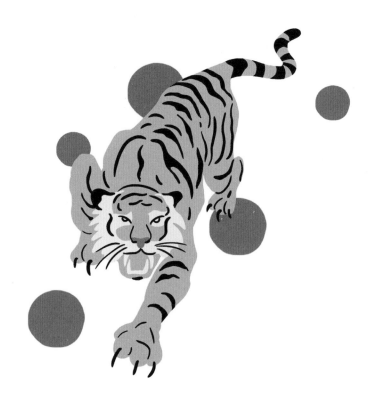

ASK DR. JENN

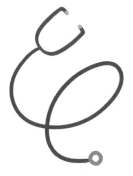

is it safe to skip my period with hormonal birth control?

There is no medical reason to have a period. In fact, the only function periods serve is to tell you you're not pregnant that month. It is absolutely safe to skip the "period week" while on hormonal birth control, by simply moving on to the next pack of birth control pills. It will not do anything untoward. This is because synthetic, external hormonal birth control keeps the inner lining of your uterus in a thin and stable state. For people with anemia, endometriosis, or really heavy periods, skipping periods can even be a miracle! So, go ahead—skip that period.

Now, if you're *not* using hormonal birth control, skipping periods can be a sign of another medical issue and you should definitely talk to your healthcare provider about that.

understanding and managing your PMS

Dr. Jenn Conti

Premenstrual syndrome, or PMS, is a term as colloquial as it is medical. It's not at all surprising that PMS has been used by the patriarchy to trivialize female behaviors, actions, and motivations. PMS is a variety of physical and behavioral changes, such as irritability, bloating, and fatigue, that happen during the latter half of the menstrual cycle, and it is totally normal. More than 90 percent of people with periods experience one or more physical or mental symptoms in the days leading up to it because of the cyclical rise and fall of the hormones that drive ovulation, progesterone being the main culprit. Progesterone is also responsible for most of the crappy symptoms of pregnancy: bloating, gastric reflux, and mood changes. This hormone is incredibly necessary but can leave you feeling pretty crummy when the levels are high.

Things start to get complicated when this normal occurrence begins interfering with your life. According to the American College of Obstetricians and Gynecologists (ACOG), the true significance of PMS emerges when symptoms like depression, pelvic pain, and anger lead to economic and/or social dysfunction. Clinically significant symptoms that interfere with daily activities affect about 8 percent of people with periods. Premenstrual dysphoric disorder (PMDD) is a more severe version of PMS that affects only about 2 percent of people with periods. In PMDD, the effects of these hormonal shifts can be so severe that people become nonfunctional or suicidal, even during the latter half of their menstrual cycles. For people who are notably affected by these changes, there are many steps they can take to improve their overall quality of life.

If you plot menstrual hormones (LH, FSH, estrogen, and progesterone) on a graph, it looks like an elaborate roller-coaster ride, climbing and falling throughout the month. The easiest and most common treatment for PMS is hormonal birth control, because it essentially levels out the natural hormonal roller coaster. By blunting the effect of the highs and lows, and keeping hormones in a steadier state, the PMS symptoms also improve. The treatment for PMDD is typically hormones plus an antidepressant/anxiolytic medication, because hormonal birth control alone typically isn't enough.

What about natural remedies for PMS? Certainly, people have been managing PMS since before modern medicine. The things that research has shown to work reliably are exercise and relaxation techniques (although typically in concert with medication). One study found women who exercised regularly had lower rates of impaired concentration and pain on a standardized menstrual distress questionnaire. However, supplements, including vitamin B6, vitamin E, chaste tree, calcium, and magnesium, don't seem to be any more effective than placebos in managing symptoms.

Acupuncture is another therapy that gets a lot of media attention for a variety of health conditions, including PMS. However, as with most Eastern medicine, it's not a one-size-fits-all approach, but rather a crafted, holistic treatment plan for each individual. It's difficult to rigorously study and academically vouch for a therapy we can't standardize across study participants. For medical professionals to officially recommend a therapy, we have to be able to prove it's both effective and safe. This means there's inevitably going to be a lot of gray area when treating conditions like PMS, because we just don't have all the research we need yet. However, when you consider the true desperation some people feel while experiencing PMS—and especially PMDD—the best management approach is one that considers all options, so long as they're safe and effective for the person.

Managing PMS in real life is as much a roller coaster as the menstrual cycle itself. Staying well informed and keeping an ongoing, open dialogue with your healthcare provider about your options is the first step toward reclaiming control of your body.

period hacks

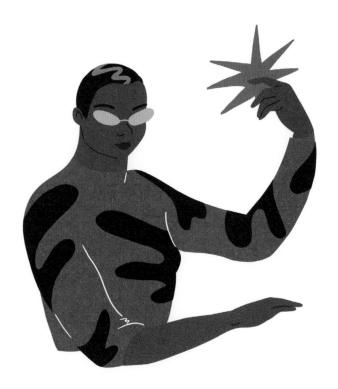

We know that *every body* is different, but just
to make things extra complicated, every person
with a period menstruates in their own unique
way. We have different cycles, different PMS
symptoms, and different period hacks. But at
least we can share our hacks! While there is no
one panacea that fits all, these are some of the
tips, tricks, and special remedies we swear by.

CBD-infused oils have proven to be the best remedy to ease my abdominal cramps and excruciating lower back aches. I like to mix a little coconut oil and lavender oil with a few drops of CBD tincture and apply topically to my sore spots. It smells incredible, and I feel immediate relief. Plus, there's something really comforting about belly rubs.

—Penda N.

I take a leaf out of my grandmother's book and go straight for the Croatian brandy, rakija. My baba swears by her potent, homemade liquor (made from fermented fruit) and uses it liberally to treat myriad aches and pains. I drink a small glass of rakija as soon as my cramps start to flare up, as well as rubbing some on my tummy. Cramps begone!

—Juliana R.

Sometimes, when my period cramps are raging, it feels like my insides have twisted up into a tight knot (I know—yuck). As soon as I feel the first jolt of pain, I turn to my heating pad, a gift my mom gave me before college that's lasted through many dorm rooms and apartments. The pad takes about 30 seconds to heat up and brings me immediate comfort when I rest it on my lower abdomen. Or, if I have the time to indulge in a more luxe, soothing activity, I'll draw a piping hot bath, bring a book, and leave my phone in my bedroom. A bath not only soothes my cramps, but gives me peace of mind. Oh, and chocolate. Lots and lots of chocolate.

—Kelsey D.

When I'm traveling (or my heating pad is "lost" under my bed somewhere), I wet a washcloth, microwave it for a minute, then put it in a plastic bag. If there's no microwave in sight, just running the rag under very hot water can do the trick too.

—Brianna F.

I go to the hottest yoga class I can find and sweat everything out. The twisting, back-bending, and stretching all make my cramps and achy body feel way better. Just need to remember to wear a slightly looser sports bra.

—Hilary F. G.

If you track your period, take your pain relief meds the night before or morning of to get ahead of the pain. I put myself on 600 mg of ibuprofen every 8 hours the day/evening leading up to my period. I usually get my period in the middle of the night, and it has really helped to control the pain.

—Leah S.

When I'm feeling especially crampy, I rub cognac on my stomach (or I drink it). Seriously, it works!

—Daniella A.

Whenever I get cramps and feel cold, I make a ginger tea with brown sugar. It's a traditional Chinese cold remedy and really heats up your abdominal area! When I'm out of brown sugar, I just boil some Coke with ginger—it does the same thing.

—Janet C.

My go-to takeout order during my period is super spicy Indian food—I get massive cravings. I'm not sure if it's because it's delicious or because of the spice, but it definitely takes my mind off of cramps!

—Laura B.

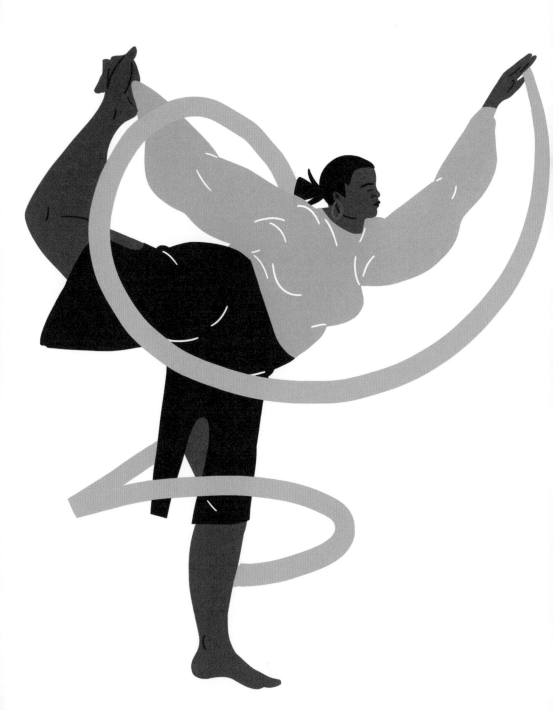

yoga poses for PMS

Arguably, there are two types of people with periods: those who feel that exercising through PMS symptoms makes them feel better, and those who would rather lie around and challenge themselves to watch an entire season of *Buffy the Vampire Slayer* without moving. For those of us who are firmly in the latter group, practicing yoga while you're PMS-ing could be a happy medium between those two. There are many reported benefits to hitting the mat, including reducing stress, boosting your mood, and best of all, getting natural period pain relief! Looking for somewhere to start? Try this simple, very beginner-friendly flow.

Remember: Skip any *asanas* (poses) that cause you more discomfort or pain. Take some time to relax into positions that work for *your* body (as you should with any yoga practice). There's no need to push yourself past your limits, especially during an already vulnerable time like menstruation. Find what works for you—even if that means keeping the TV on. There are no rules here.

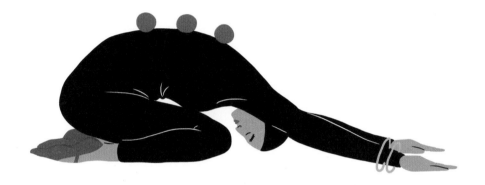

balasana (child's pose)

This natural, stress-relieving pose will gently stretch your hips, thighs, and ankles, which is why it's often the position you're told to fall into when you need a break during yoga class. You can adopt Child's Pose with your knees together or wide, whichever is more comfortable for you. For another variation that combats bloating and cramping, curl your arms over your stomach.

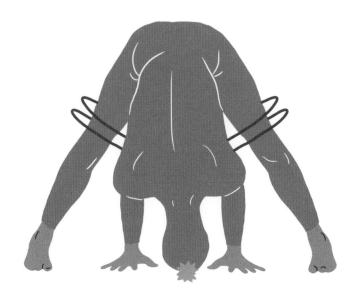

prasarita padottanasana 1 (wide-legged forward bend)

To safely enter this pose, start by standing up straight, then step your feet out sideways until they're beyond hip-width apart, wherever you feel comfortable. Slowly bend forward while propping yourself up with your hands flat on the floor (feel free to bend your knees if you need to!). Practicing inversions (when your head is below your heart) can reap many benefits, including helping you feel energized and refreshed, soothing an achy lower back, and even lowering your blood pressure.

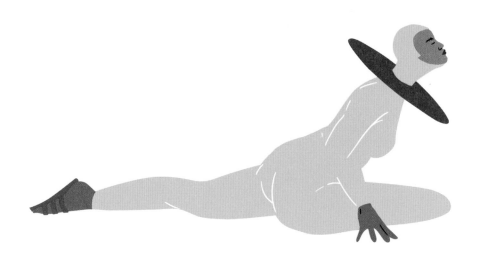

eka pada rajakapotasana variation (sleeping pigeon pose)

Ever feel so stressed while on your period that your whole body tightens up? Try this pose. Start from a plank position, then carefully bring one knee to the floor beneath your stomach, behind your wrists (be mindful of your ankle!). Slowly lower your pelvis to the floor. If you find your hips are not aligned when you settle down, you can place a block or a blanket under the hip that is raised. Once you're comfortable, walk your hands forward until you can rest your forehead down on the floor and chill out for a bit. To pick yourself back up, place your hands flat on the floor and carefully push yourself back into a plank position. Repeat with the other leg bent.

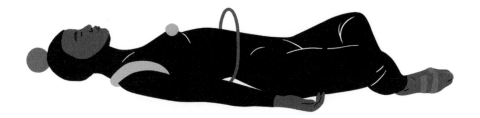

supta baddha konasana
(reclining bound angle pose)

First, lie down on your back with your knees bent.
Release your knees out to your sides, down toward your
mat, then bring the soles of your feet together. You can
prop up your knees with blocks or place a blanket under
your back (or both) if that makes you more comfortable.
You can breathe into this pose for several minutes; it's
perfect for releasing all the tension that builds up in
your hips and groin during your period.

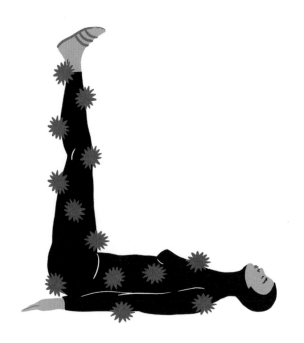

viparita karani (legs up the wall pose)

Sit yourself on the floor in front of a wall or chair, or anywhere you can prop your feet up. Lie flat on your back and walk your feet up until your body is in an "L" shape. Hang out in this position for as long as you'd like. It might take a few minutes, but any cramps you're feeling should eventually alleviate! Not only does this pose combat bloat and any tummy issues you might be having, but it's also great for giving yourself a mental breather to regain focus, especially when you're feeling your most angsty.

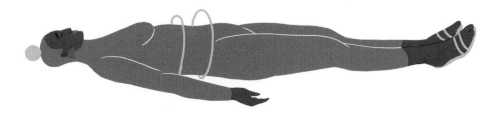

savasana (corpse pose)

It can be tempting to skip this restorative pose, but taking time to relax your muscles is an instant stress buster. Lie flat on your back, arms at your sides, and tune out any external distractions. It's totally OK if you doze off. (Hey, napping while wearing yoga pants is still yoga, right? Asking for a friend.)

Jes Tom

on learning how to insert a tampon from a GIF

I have always known about periods. Growing up, my liberal household had an open-door bathroom policy, so I believed I understood the body. Although in this way I was rather mature, in other ways I was a late bloomer. Case in point: puberty. At fourteen years old, I was gawky and ungainly, like a baby horse. Now, as a nonbinary trans adult, I am grateful for my delayed experience of puberty. But as an eighth grader—especially an eighth-grade girl (as I believed I was), I felt conflicted. On one hand, I loved being a kid. On the other, I wanted desperately to blossom into a beautiful woman and unmask the mysteries of womanhood.

Given my lifelong understanding that periods existed, I was surprised when I didn't take to menstruation with a natural grace. I thought that maybe, crossing the middle-school yard wearing a pad for the first time, I might feel like I held some deep grownup secret. But no—I felt like I was wearing a diaper. "It's a pad, isn't it?" said Janina, clocking my distress. Janina was my crass, sexually knowledgeable friend. She was the coolest. "Pads feel disgusting. I *only* use tampons." And in that moment, I decided I would too.

I decided to try my first tampon on the day of orientation for my soon-to-be high school, like debuting a new dress at a party. But when I opened the wrapper, I found something I didn't understand. I inspected the strange object: a cotton-something inside a stiff cardboard tube, with another, slimmer cardboard tube stuck into the other end, and a string threaded through. I turned it in my hands and the slimmer tube fell away, rolling across the tiles. I was baffled. Why didn't I know how to do this? As the salmon knows to swim upstream, so should I know how to insert a tampon into my vaginal canal. But this was a puzzle, and I was already running late. Never one to give up, I shoved the whole thing—cardboard tube and all—into myself and left for school.

I had chosen to attend an alternative private high school run by former hippies. This meant our orientation involved a *lot* of sitting cross-legged on the floor—an uncomfortable position when you have a three-inch long rigid tube poking out of you. Surrounded by cool and wealthy future classmates, I felt like I was carrying a secret—an embarrassing secret. I had attempted one of the rites of passage of womanhood and failed, and couldn't understand why. Maybe using a tampon was always this painful? Maybe the women joyfully playing tennis and doing yoga in tampon commercials were just grinning and bearing it?

Back home, I made a mad dash to the bathroom to free myself from the little cardboard dagger jabbing at my insides. Then I found the dark spot soaking through my underwear and into my jeans. After all that pain and discomfort, the tampon hadn't even done its job (of course, as I realized later, the actual tampon never made contact with my body). I quietly, shamefully, shelved the idea of being adult enough to use tampons, and went back to pads.

That summer, while perusing an anime chatroom, an image in someone's chat signature gave me pause. It was an animated GIF of the instructions from the side of a tampon box, showing a cross-sectioned figure inserting a tampon. The figure stuck the tip of one cardboard tube into themself, used the other tube to push the little cotton plug through, then *removed the cardboard, leaving just the cotton.* I watched it over and over, feeling a mixture of humiliation, relief, and cascading realization. Now I knew the secret—and just in time to start high school a secure, complete woman. Or so I thought.

Jes (they/them) is a New York–based actor, writer, and weird queer stand-up comic, gleefully providing the nonbinary queer Asian American radical cyborg perspective that everyone never knew they wanted.

period advice to
our younger selves

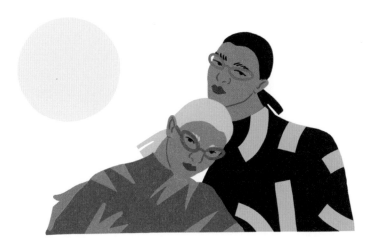

You probably made a few questionable decisions
when you were younger that you wish you could
go back in time to alter (or at least, forget). Now
that you're older and (arguably) wiser, what
period-related wisdom would you impart to
your lovably awkward adolescent self? We all
have something to learn by sharing sometimes
cringe-worthy experiences—and can hopefully
pass some of this sage-ish wisdom on to the
next generation. Check out a few tips we would
offer up if we had the chance to take a trip back
in time to visit our tween selves.

Understand that your body's hormones might go crazy with acne and insane mood swings. Just know this is temporary, nourish your skin (don't use harsh chemicals), and surround yourself with people who make you happy. There might be some strong and random sentiments that come out of nowhere, but just breathe and let them go.

—Janet C.

Hi, twelve-year-old Sam! Great job not freaking out when you got your period for the first time and Mom wasn't home. You put on a panty liner and went to the ASPCA to play with kittens like a champ. A panty liner isn't gonna cut it for much longer, though. Your period's about to get heavier. Like, way heavier. You're gonna bleed through a super tampon every 2 hours for a bit. It won't be fun, and don't let anyone (like the school nurse) tell you you're being dramatic. It's also OK to go on birth control to make your flow chill out. It doesn't mean you're a complainer or a "skank," and it won't make you gain weight (we can talk about your body image another time). Also, menstrual cups exist (look them up on the iMac)! They're way more convenient than tampons, cheaper, and better for the environment. And not gross. Anyone who tells you they're gross is not your friend.

—Sam P.

Hey girl. Guess what? Your period does not have to hurt this much! Go on birth control! OK, so it's going to take you a couple of tries to find one that doesn't make you deeply sad all the time, but it'll be worth it. (Also, while I've got you here and we're on the subject of avoiding unnecessary pain, don't cut your own bangs. You will not look like Audrey Hepburn, I promise.)

—Toni B.

My advice to my younger self would be to listen to my body and not downplay my period pain or discomfort. For many years, I convinced myself that if I talked openly about how painful my cramps were, I was being dramatic. There were days where I couldn't concentrate in class because the cramps were so intense, but I never properly advocated for myself and spoke up. I want you to know, li'l Kelsey, your pain is valid, your body deserves to be listened to, and you have permission to speak up and ask for what you want, to make your period the best experience it can be.

—Kelsey D.

You'll get your first period in a crowded public restroom, and your mom will quickly hand you a super plus tampon under the stall. But that doesn't mean it's the only option you have to manage your period. Your flow (and your body) will keep changing in all sorts of ways over time, so don't be afraid to get to know it better. What works for your mom or sisters isn't necessarily what's right for you, so try experimenting with other solutions to find the right fit. There are so many options out there!

—Rachel C.

Wash your face and change your pillowcase to avoid that pre-period zit. But also, still moisturize. And if you do get a zit (you will), keep your hands off it. *Please*. Older Hil will thank you.

—Hilary F. G.

Hey, young, curious, and dancing Penda. First things first: Your body is an amazing indicator of what's going on with you physically and emotionally. So, when you get those first pangs in your lower belly and see a few extra bumps on your face, things are definitely changing! It may take a few extra swaps of bloody underwear to realize you are becoming a woman, but trust me—it's a wonderful transformation. Bleeding can sometimes seem like it's getting in the way of you living your best life (and waking up to stained sheets is definitely the worst) but enjoy the evolution. Every period cycle is a monthly reminder that your body is incredible.

—Penda N.

Siobhán Lonergan

on what we buy when we buy period products

Most people with periods purchase products to manage their menstruation every month for decades. What do we reach for on the shelf (or add to our virtual carts), and what does it tell us about how society views our bodies and their natural processes? It might just seem like a box of tampons, but how our period products are advertised and marketed to us reflects our attitudes as a culture, and this branding can shift a person's experience of their period.

With the introduction of the first consumer period products from 1890 to 1920, marketers leveraged long-standing cultural stigma and shame to describe and sell their wares. This era of period product marketing was defined by fearmongering and portrayed the natural and healthy menstruation process as unclean, unsanitary, and unsafe. These words have deep roots, and the message—that we need separation and protection from our periods—saturated the product category for years.

Lister's Sanitary Napkins and Kotex were among the first products with branded names, which relieved the customer from having to utter the name of the unseemly item they were looking for out loud ("Kotex—Ask for us by name!"). For decades, periods remained completely hidden from period product marketing. In the 1940s, the brand Modess became a household name based on a bewildering strategy: full-page magazine spreads of fashionable ladies wearing ornate ballgowns alongside just two words of copy: "Modess because . . . " No mention of what the product is, what it's for, or even how to buy it!

Slowly, hints about what these products were actually for crept into marketing language. Through the '50s and '60s, ads promised total protection for "those days," and gave us plenty of veiled references to good times "All Through the Month!" Technical drawings of product features gave way to lavish and fantastical images of women enjoying a lifestyle of leisure and sport, with their nasty biology hidden away. Many of us think of the swinging '60s as a time for freedom of expression, and period product marketers did target freedom-loving hippies and second-wave feminists. However, this freedom didn't extend to self-acceptance, and instead meant new claims of freedom from periods. Deodorants, douches, and period products continued on a campaign to depict menstruation as a problem to be concealed and masked, rather than a natural bodily function. It wasn't until almost 100 years after the very first period products arrived on the market that the word "period" was uttered on TV, by Courtney Cox in a 1985 Tampax commercial.

But in the early aughts, backlash against unrealistic imagery in advertising set the stage for a revolution. Brands like Dove created campaigns featuring real, unretouched customers, and slowly the concept of advertising as a mirror even reached menstrual products. In 2015, Thinx brought periods front and center to the morning commute, with ads showing models wearing our eponymous period-proof underwear juxtaposed with abstract images of grapefruits and dropping eggs (representing the vagina and the menstrual cycle). Our copy declared: This is underwear "for women with periods." This wave continues, and brands are using language and images that reflect the reality of menstruation. After decades of stand-in blue liquid, in 2016 the UK brand Bodyform released an ad depicting real blood—with the tagline "No blood should hold us back." Representation matters: real periods and real experiences.

Today, magazines (and your Instagram feed) are still littered with ludicrous images of women smiling next to captions of how layers of plastic help them escape from the horror of their own bodies, but a shift is occurring. The broader focus on financial independence means more people with periods can vote with their dollars for the brands and marketing that speak to them. The advertising field is becoming more diverse than ever and placing a higher value on consumer voices to make branding decisions.

Good advertising uses universal behavioral themes to solve problems, figuring out what consumers need and addressing those issues straight on. If more advertisers listened to their customers, they'd hear them asking for authenticity above all else. And slowly, period product advertisers are realizing that secrecy, euphemisms, and whispers surrounding periods don't solve our problems; they reinforce them. But we still have our work cut out for us.

Siobhán is the Chief Brand Officer at Thinx Inc. She drives strategic brand thinking across their family of brands and ensures the seamless translation of brand strategy across all marketing, communication, and design. Currently, Siobhán lives in New York City with her husband.

menstrual hygiene through the ages

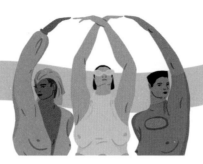

Ever wondered how people with periods dealt with things before tampons, pads, or Thinx existed? As it turns out, there isn't a lot of information about how early civilizations handled menstruation. Scribes (who were mostly men) didn't really write about periods. To be fair, our ancestors tended to menstruate much less. They started their flows in their late teens, spent more time pregnant or breastfeeding, hit menopause earlier, and died earlier. (Rough.) From what we do know, it seems like they used wool, cotton lint wrapped around splinters of wood (ouch?!), and whatever else was lying around to fashion pads and tampons on the fly. Check out how some other menstrual innovations came to be.

LONG, LONG AGO

One of the oldest period products on record is actually still used today: the sponge. Nope, not the dish sponge behind your sink faucet you probably should've changed 7 months ago, but sea sponges, from the actual sea. These sponges (once inserted) absorbed menstrual blood and held sperm-killing liquids.

3100 BC

Ancient Egyptians fashioned tampons out of softened papyrus and grass before cotton became the preferred material in the Roman era. They also found some alternative uses for menstrual blood, like incorporating it into spell casting (cool!). Sometimes, this involved drinking it (less cool!).

FIFTH TO FIFTEENTH CENTURIES

During the Middle Ages, layered strips of cloth were the period product of choice. This practice continued into the early nineteenth century, when the phrase "on the rag" became a thing. That's not to say they couldn't get crafty: One remedy for heavy periods involved wearing burnt toad ashes in a pouch near your vagina. Let's assume that didn't work too well.

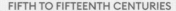

1896

Johnson & Johnson released Lister's Towels (a nod to surgeon Dr. Joseph Lister), the first commercially available pads in the United States. Due to modest turn-of-the-century sensibilities, the ads had to be vague; thus, they had a very limited reach. Menstruation was still too taboo of a subject for the product to sell.

1920

Kotex introduced an innovation first discovered by French nurses during WWI: Cellulose, a cotton-acrylic blend used for bandages, absorbed blood way better than plain old cotton. Kotex's big Don Draper–level idea was to showcase nurses in their ads. Since talking about your period was still verboten, period product marketers at this time got smart in helping shoppers obtain their products. Some asked retailers to place the products on counters, with coin boxes next to them, so shoppers could pay for their purchases discreetly. Another company advertised a "silent coupon" to hand to a clerk that said, "One box of [product], please." No embarrassing talking required!

1929

The first official tampon hit the scene thanks to Dr. Earle C. Haas, a doctor from Colorado. Haas's wife hated pads, and he really came through with an alternative. Haas's tampons were made of thick cotton and featured a cardboard applicator.

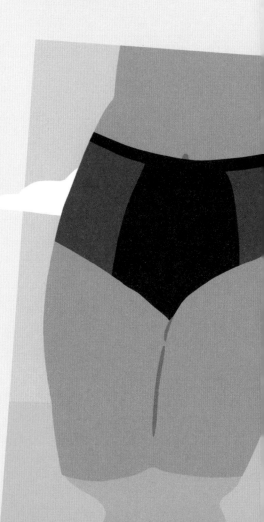

1936

Denver businesswoman Gertrude Tendrich, who bought the tampon patent in 1933, founded the Tampax company. The backlash to commercial tampons was swift. People were not into the idea of women touching themselves in any way (*eye roll*) and were convinced tampons could break a virgin's hymen (*double eye roll*).

1937

Actress Leona Chalmers invented the menstrual cup—and considering the fuss over girls putting in tampons, it should not come as a shock that the cup did not fly with many audiences either. However, the menstrual cup has maintained a small but loyal following through the decades and has been enjoying a resurgence in recent years.

1956

If you're wondering how people kept their pads in place before adhesive, meet the sanitary belt, which held pads in place with, well, a belt. Mary Beatrice Davidson Kenner (a badass you've probably never heard of) patented the belt, but her initial investors backed out when they found out she was a Black woman.

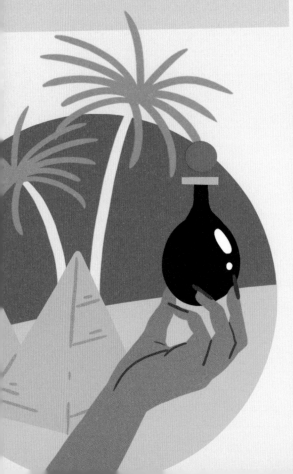

1975

Procter & Gamble introduced Rely, advertised as tampons you could wear for the length of an entire period. If that sounds too good to be true, that's because it was. It was revealed that the synthetic materials used to make Rely changed a woman's vaginal pH and acted like the agar in a petri dish, two factors that encouraged bacterial growth and infection. After 812 reported cases of toxic shock syndrome, Rely was taken off shelves. Today, there is still no law that requires tampons to list their materials on their boxes, which is why our mothers will obsessively warn us about keeping our tampons in too long for the remainder of eternity.

2013

Thinx, underwear that absorbs your period, was invented. Thinx was the first "new" menstrual care product to hit the market since the menstrual cup. (If you've been following along, you'll remember that was nearly 80 years previous!)

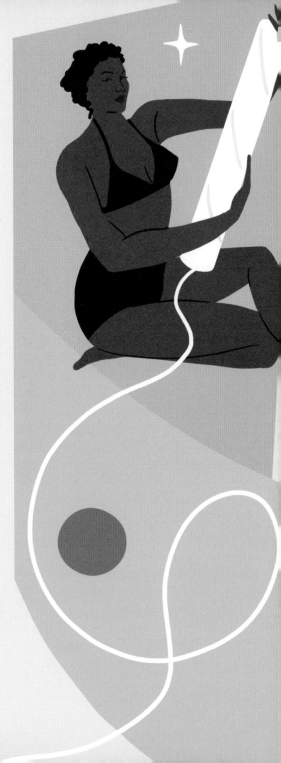

we need to talk about period poverty

Quick question—would you ever bring your own toilet paper into a bathroom? It's probably safe to say your answer is no. So why aren't period products considered basic necessities in the same way? Periods are a natural function of the human body. Yet, in many countries, tampons and pads are often classified as luxury items, rendering them inaccessible to those who need them the most.

This might not seem like a big deal, but access to period products determines a person's freedom to work, study, and move about the world with basic dignity. Millions of people around the world live in period poverty, unable to afford basic necessities to manage their menstruation. People who don't have access to (or enough of) these products often resort to wearing tampons and pads for longer than recommended, which puts them at higher risk for cervical cancer, or infections like toxic shock syndrome.

the period taboo

The United Nations officially declared menstrual hygiene a public health issue in 2014, but the period taboo has allowed this human rights crisis to thrive. In 2018, a network of Chicago charter schools came under fire for allowing their menstruating students to tie sweatshirts around their waists to hide visible blood-stains rather than permitting them to take regular bath-room breaks—as if that solves the problem of children sitting in uncomfortable, over-filled period products all day, or stops the culture of shame that stigmatizes those who menstruate. And in rural Nepal, women are frequently banished from their homes every month to "menstrual huts" where conditions are sometimes fatal.

Period poverty is devastating, and the consequences can be serious. It's time to give this issue the attention it deserves, especially in areas where we can make tan-gible steps toward change.

our fight for menstrual equity

In 2018, Thinx Inc. launched its first national grassroots campaign, United for Access, alongside PERIOD, the world's largest youth-run nonprofit dedicated to chang-ing the conversation around periods and providing care to those in need. Our first initiative was to circulate petitions in cities across the country demanding that every student in the United States—from grade school through college—has free and easy access to period products. (No one should have to miss out on an educa-tion because of their period!)

actions you can take today

If there's one thing we learned from our inaugural campaign, it's that when it comes to menstrual equity, actions on a local and grassroots level can be incredibly influential. That makes it easy for anyone (here's lookin' at you, kid!) to take actionable, often simple steps toward advocating for people with periods in their own communities.

1. As of 2019, 35 states tax period products. If you're in one of these states, figure out who your reps are, put them on speed dial, and call them to advocate for banishing the "tampon tax."

2. Advocate for free and accessible period products in your community's public restrooms. Our institutions should be serving *us*, and we have the power to initiate change; approaching PTAs and student boards at local schools with a petition and a plan is a good place to start. No one's education should be limited by access to necessities!

3. Call up your friends and host a period kit packing party! Reach out to local organizations for help locating groups that accept donations. A couple cycles' worth of tampons and pads could make such a difference for someone who lacks access to these products. (Be mindful when donating reusable products like cups and Thinx; the recipient will need reliable access to water, changing, and cleaning facilities in order to use those products safely.)

4. Be #periodproud. It can be tough to advocate for an issue no one wants to talk about. Do your part to dismantle any internal stigma you may still carry about menstruating, and then tell the world! OK, you don't have to go that far, but if you're up for it, try not to overtly conceal your period or how you're managing it, especially with people who don't have a period. (No one will combust if they see a tampon, we promise.)

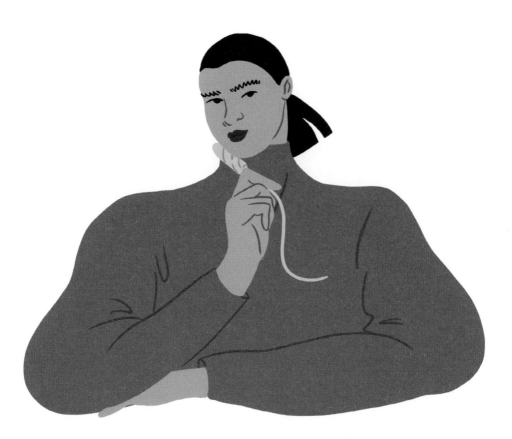

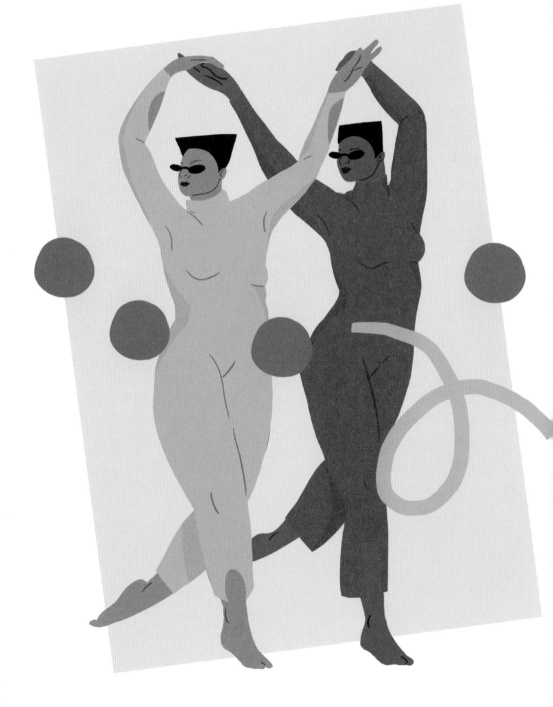

irregular periods (and when to call your gyno)

First things first: Let's do away with the idea that irregular, abnormal, or different always equals bad. Remember, once upon a time people thought ladies wearing pants was weird too! That said, there is such a thing as a typical period for you, and keeping tabs on your flow is important. Changes in your cycle might mean absolutely nothing, or they might be your body's way of signaling that something bigger is going on.

Theoretically, your period should show up every 21 to 35 days, and last anywhere from 2 to 7 days (where do we sign up for the 48-hour flow?). Since there are tons of factors that can influence your cycle, having an irregular period is actually an umbrella term for a few different scenarios.

At opposite ends of the irregular period spectrum are amenorrhea, when your period is MIA for at least 3 to 6 months, and menorrhagia, when you have abnormally heavy or prolonged bleeding (going through more than one tampon or pad an hour for hours on end, periods lasting longer than 8 days, etc.). In the middle is variations in your period month to month—whether it's showing up late, you're spotting in between cycles, or it's lighter or heavier than usual.

Most people with periods don't menstruate on a strict calendar, but if you've been like clockwork for a while and your period schedule or blood volume is suddenly thrown, it's a good idea to look into potential causes.

pregnancy

If you're having reproductive sex and your period hasn't shown up lately, it's possible that you're pregnant. A standard stick test can usually tell you if you're pregnant as early as 2 weeks after conception, so it's worth investing in the test or a trip to a Planned Parenthood clinic or other organization that can help you figure it out for free.

NOTE: Watch out for crisis pregnancy centers. These are fake women's clinics; they might give you a free pregnancy test, but many of these groups use scare tactics to enforce an underlying anti-abortion agenda. Seek advice from a neutral medical professional who will inform you about *all* your options—including parenting, adoption, and abortion—if your test is positive.

Also, while we're talking about pregnancy: No matter what the internet tells you, it's not medically possible to menstruate while you're pregnant. Some people spot early on in their pregnancy, which usually looks like light pink or dark brown discharge. But bleeding enough to fill any menstrual product is a sign that you're either not pregnant, you're miscarrying, or you're having a complication with the pregnancy—it's worth a call to your doctor.

stress

Your mental state does affect your bodily health. If your period is irregular or not showing up at all (and you're not pregnant), it might be that everyday stress—both emotional (depression, anxiety) and physical (rapid weight gain or loss, illness)—is taking a bigger toll on your body than you realize. Your reproductive system is run by two hormones: estrogen and progesterone. When you get super stressed out, the hypothalamus and pituitary glands in your brain can have a harder time regulating the natural rhythm of your reproductive hormones, which can cause spotting, a late or skipped period, or extra-intense PMS symptoms.

If you think stress might be the culprit (and even if you don't) make sure you prioritize relaxation and self-care. It looks different for everybody, so figure out what *you* need to unwind. Giving yourself some extra TLC and having a chat about your symptoms with your gyno are two important steps in getting your period back on track.

perimenopause and other hormonal fluctuations

Hormonal ups and downs are a totally normal part of being human (middle school, anybody?), but it's a pretty common misconception that puberty has the only big shift in hormones. During perimenopause, the body's estrogen production gradually decreases, and the lining of the uterus thins. It may all be natural, but perimenopause can make your period do pretty wild things. For some, periods come to a dramatic halt, and others will see their period gradually peter out over time. But most perimenopausal people experience some unpredictability, from spotting, to shorter cycles, to unexpectedly heavy or light flows.

hormonal contraception

If you've just started taking the pill, the patch, the ring, or any other form of hormonal contraception, it's pretty normal to experience some spotting as your body adjusts, especially in the first 3 months or so. That said, missing a pill or two, even after years of being on birth control, can cause some unexpected bleeding between cycles. Since birth control pills deliver a steady stream of hormones to your system, a sudden break or adjustment in your birth control can trick your uterus into thinking it's time to shed its lining (no matter how inconvenient that might be during your beach vacay).

underlying health issues

If you can rule out any of the above scenarios as causes, irregular periods could also be a symptom of undetected health issues. Fibroids, endometriosis, polycystic ovary syndrome (PCOS), and certain STIs are just a few medical conditions that can affect your flow. If your period is heavier than normal or comes with serious pain (meaning way more than your standard period cramps), it's definitely worth a chat with your doctor to see if something else is going on.

No matter your symptoms, irregular periods are as good a reason as any to schedule your next gyno visit. Your doctor can help you decipher your symptoms and work with you to get to the bottom of what's really going on. After all, the more you know and understand your bod, the better you can care for it.

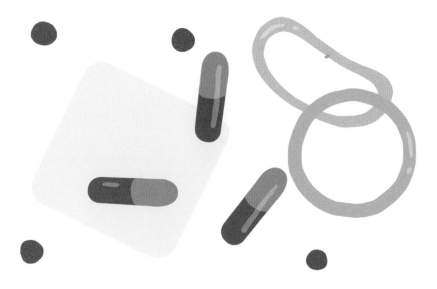

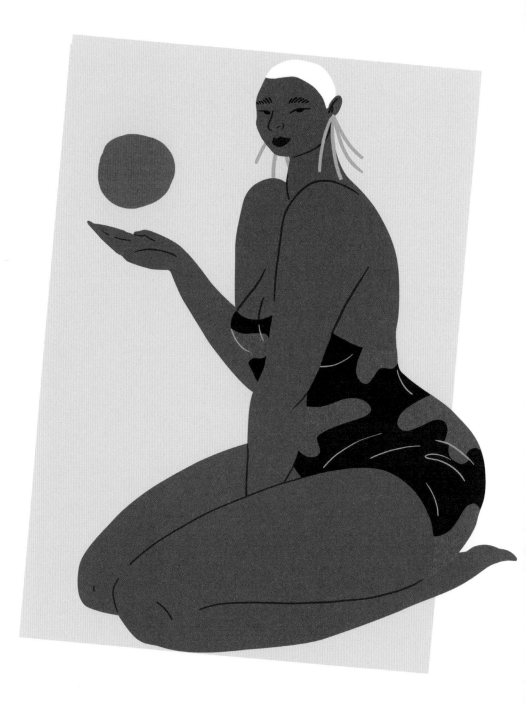

making the case for period sex

For some people with periods, sex during their flow is the go-to remedy for uncomfortable symptoms like cramps or anxiety. But for others, even the idea of period sex is saddled with all kinds of negative thoughts and emotions: shame, fear, disgust, or stress about messy sheets. We can thank patriarchy for period shame in all its shapes and forms—it's pervasive and can be hard to shake. No matter what you've heard, the truth is that period sex is fun, natural, and even healthy. Yes, it can get a little messy, but it's nothing a rinse cycle can't handle, and the benefits make doing an extra load of laundry a pretty fair trade.

Studies show that sex—whether it's a solo or partnered event—can reduce uncomfortable PMS symptoms and provide overwhelmingly positive health effects.

fewer headaches

If migraines go hand in hand with your flow, you'll be happy to know that having more sex can help you out. Your brain produces all kinds of feel-good chemicals when you're doin' it, like dopamine and oxytocin—chemicals that can reduce the effects of stress hormones like cortisol in your body, which, in turn, can help relax your mind and stave off headaches before they take hold.

better mood

Again, you can thank those feel-good chemicals for giving sex its generous benefits. During an orgasm, your body releases endorphins, which are neurotransmitters often associated with pleasurable activities, like eating, drinking, and relaxing. (BTW, sex can be a great mood booster any time of the month, not just during your period.)

cramp and pain alleviation

When you climax, blood flow to your pelvic area increases and the uterine muscles contract, while your brain releases those feel-good and pain-relieving chemicals. Think of orgasms as your body's built-in ibuprofen supply for that time of the month.

bigger, better orgasms

Arguably, the ultimate possible upside of having period sex is the notion that some people feel increased genital sensation during this part of the cycle. It's true that hormonal fluctuations during your period can change sexual desire and bodily response, but the jury is still out on whether or not science can support this claim. All you can do is try it yourself to see if it's true! Either way, your flow can serve as a natural lubricant to make penetrative sex more pleasurable. (But let's not forget—penetrative sex isn't the only way to do it.)

Whether you're on your period or not, it's always important to practice safe sex and use whatever birth control works best for you if you aren't trying to get fertilized—menstrual blood allegedly has many super-powers, but STI protection and contraception aren't on the list.

Stigmas surrounding periods and period sex can be intense (self-scrutiny and good old shame, for example), but that doesn't mean the process of undoing them can't also be fun. Check out our suggestions for positions to try if you're ready to kick things off with a *bang*.

spooning

Cramps, bloating, and other super fun and glamorous symptoms can make literally any physical activity feel impossible during your period. Spooning is a comfy, intimate, and low-impact way to get busy without having to do too much. Plus, it's the perfect position if your boobs are feeling especially tender.

doggie style

Try modifying this position by lying flat on your stomach to ease tension from cramps. Bonus: Lots of people say doggie style is the best position for G-spot stimulation (see page 145 for more on the mythical G-spot).

missionary

On heavier flow days, doing missionary position (with your pelvis tilted slightly up) can minimize leaks. Try placing a pillow underneath your pelvis or putting your legs on your partner's shoulders. Protect those high-thread-count sheets!

in the shower

This one's more of an environment than a position, so feel free to get creative with the details (and if you're worried about things getting too slippery, it's definitely worth investing in one of those sticky mats for some added traction). No matter how you do it, sex in the shower is a great way to mix things up. The best part? No mess!

There's no right or wrong way to give period sex a test drive—it's important to do what feels right for you and move at your own pace. It might take a few tries before you feel fully comfortable, or you may find that period sex just isn't for you! That's OK too. The only person who gets to choose what to do with your body is you.

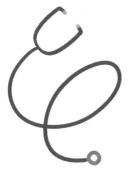

Roxane Gay
on learning how to bleed

By the time I was fourteen, I was well versed in the young adolescent literary canon inspired mostly by Judy Blume (*Are You There God? It's Me, Margaret*, and *Forever*), Francine Pascal (*Sweet Valley High*), and Emily Chase (*The Girls of Canby Hall*). These books taught me many things, not the least of which is that men name their cocks. These books also gave me a general idea of what it meant to get my period, and by general I mean vague and not at all accurate or realistic. I knew there would be pain involved, perhaps extreme pain that would require me to repose, on a bed, with the back of my hand pressed to my forehead. There would be heating pads and dramatic mood swings.

These are things I learned about periods from disreputable sources (which means, of course, that I believed them fervently):

A man could smell that you were on your period when you sat next to him.

You couldn't have sex on your period.

Having your period made you dirty.

You couldn't get pregnant while on your period.

You didn't have your period if you went on birth control.

You could be eaten by a bear if you went camping while on your period.

Women often have heart-warming stories of the day they got their period, stories where their female family members gathered round and helped them celebrate their rising womanhood. I've heard stories of bleeding parties and touching moments in the bathroom over a box of Tam-pax or Stayfree Maxi Pads. My mother always told me to enjoy my period-free days, that bleeding was a curse, and as such, I knew menstruating was not going to be celebrated in my family.

I got my period in the middle of the night, early during my sophomore year of high school. I was alone in a dormitory at a New England boarding school, in the dimly lit bathroom, staring at the metal plate cov-ering the drain near my toes. The drain plate fascinated me because it bore the last name of one of my classmates. I had

known he was rich, but had not realized he was "in bathrooms all over the world" rich. Water was dripping from a leaky faucet. It was a scene out of a bad horror movie. I was certain a serial killer would, at any moment, force his way into the bathroom to take me—young, ripe, nubile—to his lair. Blood would be involved. Then, I looked down and blood was, indeed, involved.

There was a Woolworth's in town so I walked downtown and stalked the feminine hygiene aisle, trying to make sense of the various kinds of pads and tampons, and I made a few best guesses as to which products I would need. Back in my dorm room, I read each instructional pamphlet carefully, and before long I had taught myself to manage my period. I am not at all sure why I didn't ask my mother for help, but we never talked about our bodies, and I suppose I assumed that this was some-thing I was going to have to handle independently, the way I tried to handle everything else.

My high school was good at many things—academics, grooming the sons and daughters of privilege for lives of continued good fortune, exposing students to culture, providing access to high-quality drugs—the usual things. My high school was very bad at preparing students for the basics of adolescence. They treated us like we were simply adults who hadn't yet graduated from high school. The powers that be didn't worry over the little details like puberty, emotional immaturity, and the stupidity that is unavoidable between the ages of 13 and 19. We got free condoms during special sex education events, and there was the unwritten but oft-spoken rule about one free abortion per female student. However, there was no functional system in place for helping young women learn about how to deal with their periods. The assumption, I think, was that we would learn about how to deal with our "female troubles" from other girls in the dorms or our mothers or *Seventeen* magazine. Ultimately, our blood was not on their hands. It was on our own.

It often seems like the world doesn't know how to deal with women. Bleeding at boarding school (as within many other institutions) reflects larger societal attitudes toward women, their bodies, and the natural functions of those bodies. At my school, it was acknowledged that we were sexual beings who could get pregnant, but the changes that made these things possible were ignored. What do we do with the bleeding woman? How do we acknowledge her fertility? How do we help confused, young women deal with the facts of life? These are questions that many years ago, my boarding school was unable to answer. I would not be surprised to learn that these questions are still going unanswered. Institutions are often male in character. It is not surprising, then, that they cannot deal with the awkwardness, messiness, and reality of menstruation. In the end, I learned how to bleed through trial and error, through the lore I had gleaned from pop culture, and from my own body. I also learned there is a great deal of value in what institutions and the patriarchy tend to dismiss.

Roxane's writing appears in *Best American Mystery Stories 2014*, *Best American Short Stories 2012*, *Best Sex Writing 2012*, *A Public Space*, *McSweeney's*, *Tin House*, *Oxford American*, *American Short Fiction*, *Virginia Quarterly Review*, and many other publications. She is a contributing opinion writer for the *New York Times*, and the author of *Ayiti*, *An Untamed State*, and the *New York Times* bestsellers *Bad Feminist*, *Difficult Women*, *Hunger*, and *Not That Bad*. Roxane has several books forthcoming, and is also at work on television and film projects.

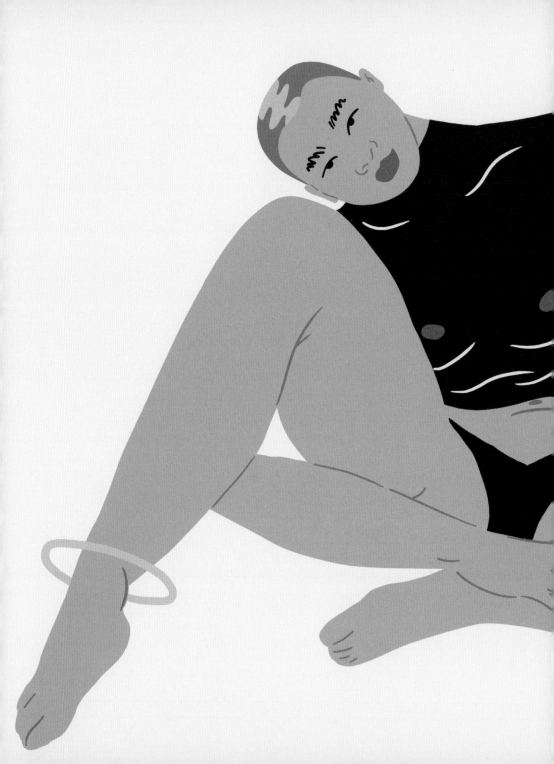

vaginal health

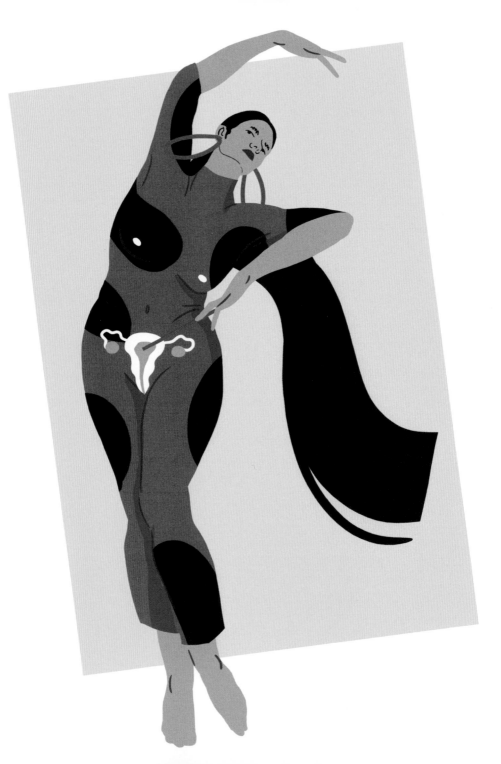

vaginal anatomy

You probably think you know where your vagina is . . . but do you? Not to be all "Well actually," but even though the term "vagina" is colloquially used to describe the whole genital area, the correct term is "vulva." The vulva includes everything down there: the clitoris, the labia, the pubic mound, and the holes for the urethra and the vagina. The vagina is actually the muscular tunnel between the vulva and the cervix.

Here's an anatomy crash course:

The cervix is a donut-shaped opening that connects the vagina to the uterus. The cervix shape and location changes depending on the time of the menstrual cycle: During a period, the cervix is lower in the body and more open than other times of the cycle. The consistency of the mucus it secretes (egg white–like or clear and sticky) tells you a lot about where you are in your cycle.

Above the cervix is the uterus—the fist-sized organ where an egg, if fertilized, will implant and grow into a fetus. The uterus is lined with a thick layer of blood, tissue, and nutrients, which will help nourish a fetus if necessary. If there is no pregnancy, the uterus sheds this lining every 28 days or so, and a new one grows. This, of course, is the menstrual period.

The fallopian tubes attach to the uterus and open up to the ovaries, where ova (human egg cells) live and grow. Ovaries serve a double function: They are also an endocrine gland that secretes hormones. If sperm is present in the fallopian tubes from sex or artificial insemination, the ovum may unite with the sperm there and become fertilized before traveling down and attaching to the wall of the uterus. These internal reproductive organs are very goal-oriented: Their singular mission is to prepare for and manage pregnancy.

The external portion, called the vulva, has several different jobs. The inner and outer labia are essentially folds of skin that act like a barrier against infection and external irritants. Everyone's labia are different: They can be long, short, or uneven lengths, and it's all normal. Labia might also be a different skin color than the surrounding area. Outer labia (labia majora) are often covered in pubic hair after puberty, unless the hair is removed. Inner labia (labia minora) tend to be moister and a different skin texture than the outer labia. After menopause, lack of estrogen can sometimes fuse these two layers together in a process called labial agglutination (what?!).

The labia protect two openings into the body: the ure-thral opening (where pee comes out) and the vaginal opening. The urethral opening connects the urethra to the bladder, and has nothing to do with the reproductive system, other than that it's pretty darn close to it—hence the old adage "pee after sex," so that bacteria that's been mushed around from the vagina and anus during sex doesn't crawl up the urethra and give you a UTI. The vaginal opening leads to—you guessed it—the vagina, and it's where a penis, finger, tampon, etc. goes in, and period blood and babies come out. The hymen is a thin, donut, semicircle or half-moon shaped membrane present just above the vaginal opening at birth. Its presence, absence, and general condition is also the focus of way too much attention by people without one (and for absolutely no sound medical reason). But more on that later.

The most unique part of the external anatomy is the clitoris. This organ is unlike any other, because its sole purpose is to provide sexual pleasure. Up until recently, we thought the clitoris was just the small, internal spot located above the urethra, but thanks to a 2009 report by Dr. Odile Buisson and Dr. Pierre Foldés, we now know that is literally the tip of the clitoral iceberg. The internal clitoris is a wishbone-shaped structure that has "branches" reaching through the pelvic area and surrounding the vagina. Just the exposed area contains thousands of nerve endings, making it extremely sensitive. Many people with this anatomy need some stimulation of the clitoris during sex in order to have an orgasm.

These descriptions represent typical anatomy, but these organs can vary widely in appearance and function beyond the cosmetic differences we've mentioned already. For example, nearly 2 percent of the population is born intersex, meaning they can have some combination of typically male and typically female sex characteristics. However, an intersex person might not have outwardly different genitalia, but possess nontypical chromosomal pairs. Traditionally, doctors and parents often choose to perform surgery on a child born intersex in order to more closely align the child's body with typical male or female genitalia. A more modern approach encourages parents to wait until the child is older to let them develop their identity. Reproductive anatomy can also be changed through hormone therapy or surgery that aims to align a person's body with their gender identity. Taking testosterone, for example, often causes the clitoris to grow and elongate a bit.

Self-exploration with a mirror, masturbation, and talking with a trusted healthcare provider and your sexual partners are all important aspects of getting to know your unique body.

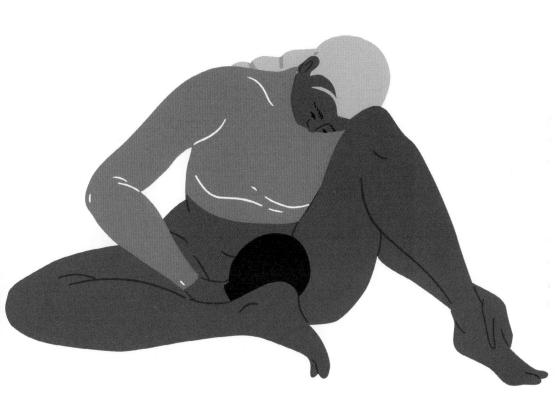

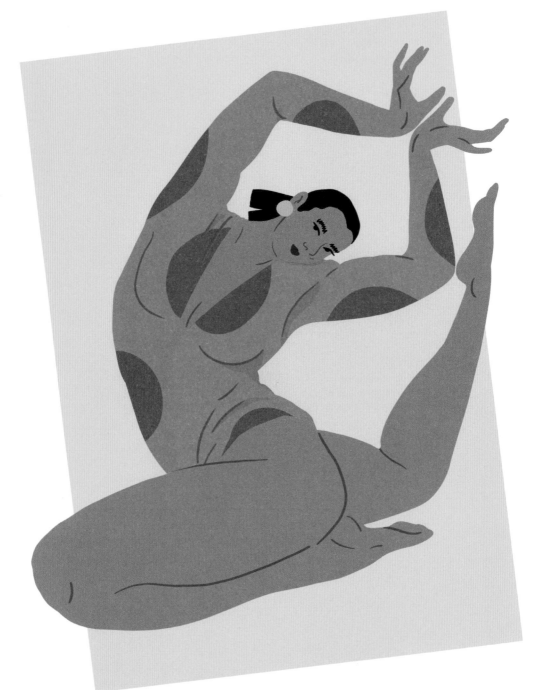

the hymen: a misunderstood membrane

Nothing reveals the general confusion that surrounds vaginal anatomy more clearly than googling "hymen." You've probably heard the hymen described in one of several ways: a barrier, some kind of wall, or, at the very least, breakable. This makes sense when you think about its historical significance (and current importance in many parts of the world) in "proving" a woman's sexual purity. The importance tied to female virginity has contributed to the widespread misinformation about hymens, and unfortunately, it's difficult to start from scratch when it comes to a topic that has been so ill-defined for centuries, but we'll do our best to separate the facts from the misconceptions.

all hymens are not created equal

Hymens are unique to each individual, similar to the way other body parts vary in size and shape: Some are thin and others are more elastic. It's possible that over time the hymen has evolved to work as a barrier to prevent vaginal infections. The ambiguity surrounding its exact purpose has allowed people to define it in a narrative that best suits their agendas. We venture an educated guess that most of the people presenting oppressive narratives don't have vaginas themselves.

Sometimes people are born with hymens that cover more of the vaginal opening than is healthy. Here are three common hymenal variants:

- Imperforate: The membrane completely covers the vaginal opening (occurs in approximately 1 out of every 1,000 people born with a vagina).

- Microperforate: Similar to an imperforate hymen, but with a smaller-than-normal (a "micro") opening to the vagina.

- Septate: An extra band of tissue creates two small vaginal openings instead of one.

Depending on the size and shape of the hymen, it could be difficult or even impossible to insert tampons or have penetrative sex. If period blood can't exit the body because the hymen blocks the opening, pain and swelling can occur. The good news is that any of these conditions can be easily corrected with an outpatient procedure when diagnosed.

the virginity fraud

If you're still wondering whether hymens and the concept of virginity have any valid relation, look up the amazing TED Talk "The Virginity Fraud" by Dr. Nina Dølvik Brochmann and Ellen Støkken Dahl. In it, they debunk the two common myths about hymens that are used to "prove" virginity: one, hymens break and bleed after sex, and two, when the hymen "breaks," it's radically altered or disappears.

For the purposes of clarity, a virgin is traditionally defined as someone who has not engaged in hetero penis-in-vagina sex. Considering how different people's hymens can be, it's virtually impossible to simply look at the condition of someone's hymen and prove whether or not they've had sex. A hymen can stretch or tear after sex, but it can also be altered by a number of nonsexual activities, including exercise, tampon use, and medical exams, as well as by masturbation. In some cases, hymens also aren't altered at all—studies have even reported women going into labor with their hymens still intact.

As doctors Brochmann and Dahl conclude in their talk, if some people's hymens don't break or bleed, and hymens can tear or naturally wear away through any number of activities besides sex, then there just isn't a conclusive way to "prove" virginity that's accurate for every person with a vagina.

While hymens might help prevent vaginal infections, no one talks about that function. Hymens are still assigned the very important role of "virginity marker" worldwide, to varying degrees of harm. The misplaced importance society has placed upon hymens has caused everything from inconvenience to outright danger to women and other people with vaginas. Hymen reconstruction surgery or "revirginization" is a very real, potentially scary thing. (Bonus scary fact: There's also a whole market for blood capsules you can use to create the illusion of a torn hymen.)

On a more practical level, the misconception that your hymen will tear, bleed, and cause you pain is also why a lot of people simply deal with having painful intercourse when they're young, or just starting to have sex. Painful sex is *not* normal, y'all. A little discomfort is to be expected, but know your body, and know that you're allowed to enjoy sex as slowly and gently as you want.

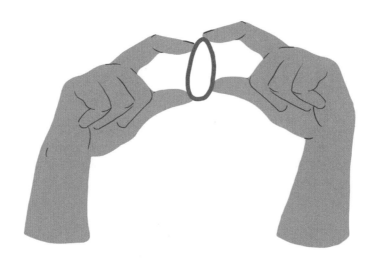

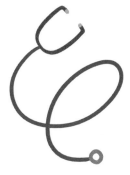

what are some ways to make first-time sex less uncomfortable?

The first time is always going to be a little nerve-racking, but pain should not be assumed inevitable.

1. Good communication is key. It sets the foundation for feeling comfortable, respected, and safe, all of which are vital components of enjoyable sex. If you know you're ready but you're feeling nervous, talk about it—before, during, and after!

2. Vaginal lubrication is the key to comfortable sex. Moistness is produced by your vagina when you're turned on, but if you're a little nervous (or just need a little extra), lube should be your best friend. Just remember to use a water- or silicone-based lube if you're using a condom; anything else could interfere with the efficacy of the condom.

3. Go slow. There's no rush, especially when you're learning to navigate sex and what you enjoy.

Blair Imani

on why virginity is bullsh*t

While it is referenced in religious texts, classical literature, and a few uncomfortable discussions in doctors' offices, many of us will be relieved to know that virginity (like many human constructs) simply does not exist. The idea that vaginal penetration fundamentally changes your worth as a human being is medically inaccurate and completely rooted in patriarchy, heteronormativity, and of course, sexism.

The construct of virginity has plagued the lives of pretty much everyone. Feminine individuals are defined by their relationships to masculine bodies. People with penises are tasked with harvesting virginities from the moment they're able to achieve an erection. People with vaginas are expected to remain pure and untouched, only able to indulge in unexplored sexual proclivities after wearing a white gown at a lavish and expensive ceremony assuring all of their relatives and loved ones that their virginity has been maintained. According to some particularly harmful folklore, people with vaginas are like cucumbers before they are penetrated, becoming foul (though some would say more delicious) pickles afterward, and remaining so until their deaths.

I was fortunate to grow up removed from these fantasies. When I told my mother the Catholic girls' school I had attended would be holding a purity ring ceremony, she forbade me from participating. My mother taught me from a very young age that the concept of sexual purity was created to maintain patriarchal control over anyone with a vagina. But even though I had this radical (and honestly, extremely accurate) upbringing at home, I was still exposed to medically inaccurate sexual education courses. I remember feeling so lost when a religious leader told me and an auditorium full of other teenagers that virgin women are like unlit candles— and who would want to buy a candle that has already been lit? Now that I am older and wiser, I know relationships are not about commerce and flames, but that metaphor stuck with me for a long time.

Here's what I wish I could've told myself (and all those other kids in the auditorium, too): Your opinion and feelings on how you view and accept your own body are yours and yours alone. If you're like my mother and believe sex is something that is amazing and important and good, then I wish you all of the amazing sex you can accommodate in your life. If you believe the first time you have sex should be special and sacred, then I wish you the most special and sacred experience that has ever transpired. If you're like me and you did not get to choose when this first time happened—because we live in a rape culture—be assured that your worth has nothing to do with the penetrative acts of an abusive body.

Every day, our bodies create new cells. We will continue to regenerate throughout our lifetime—so will our sexual organs. More than that, we must understand that virginity is an idea formulated eons ago by people concerned with policing bodies with vaginas. As a society, we must reflect on the ways medically inaccurate sex education that is imbued with archaic definitions of human experiences (like the first time a person has sex) are harmful and detrimental to adolescent development and public health. Young people are forced to become obsessed with penetration when they should be learning about consent, STI prevention, and prophylactics.

We must combat the bullsh*t around virginity and replace it with inclusive, healthy, and medically accurate sex education. We must do this because virginity simply does not exist.

Blair is a writer, mental health advocate, and historian living at the intersections of Black, Queer, and Muslim identities. In addition to being a public speaker, Blair is the author of *Modern HERstory: Stories of Women and Nonbinary People Rewriting History* (2018) and *Making Our Way Home: The Great Migration and the Black American Dream* (2020). She is also the official ambassador of Muslims for Progressive Values, one of the oldest progressive Muslim organizations to support the LGBTQ+ community.

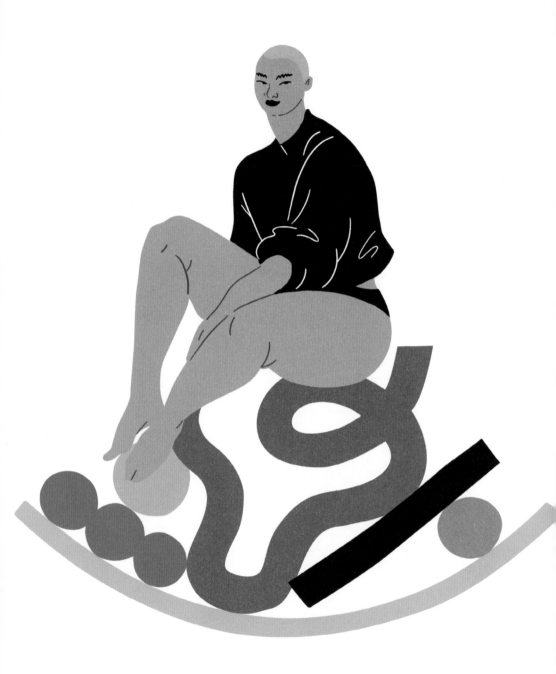

everything you should know about your pelvic floor

Many women's health issues are shrouded in mystery, and the pelvic floor might be the most mysterious of them all. That's partly because of the widespread misconception that pelvic floor health only matters for people of a certain age, or after childbirth. The truth is, taking care of your floor can help prevent many conditions from developing down the line, especially sensitive issues like bladder leaks, constipation, or pain during sex.

So, what is your pelvic floor? The simplest explanation is that it's kind of like a hammock for your organs, extending from your pubic bone to your tailbone, that cradles your insides every time you breathe. That seems pretty straightforward, but it's actually a pretty complex system of muscles (forty-five muscles connected to your pelvis!) that has three main jobs:

1. Waste elimination: It controls the closing and opening of your bowel and bladder.

2. Organ support: It ensures the organs don't literally fall out of your body (but if you experience pelvic organ prolapse, you have options).

3. Sexual appreciation: Contractions during orgasm are all thanks to your pelvic floor muscles.

Because your pelvic floor has so many big responsibilities, when something is off, it can present in a variety of ways: Incontinence, painful sex, lower back pain, hip pain, and constipation are just a few. Symptoms of pelvic floor dysfunction are less than fun, so we're all for taking care of your floor. There are a few different ways to give it some TLC, and the more methods you try out, the better off you'll be.

be mindful of your breath

Every time you inhale, your diaphragm expands and puts pressure on all of the organs that sit beneath it. It's the job of your pelvic floor muscles to react to that pressure by offering your insides some much-needed support. If your diaphragm doesn't expand fully or properly during most of your 20,000 breaths throughout the day, it can throw off your internal pressure system and put too much pressure on your pelvic floor to respond—which explains why you might leak a little pee doing jumping jacks, coughing, or a having a hearty laugh.

pay attention to your fiber intake

When it comes to pelvic floor health, what you eat plays a huge role in helping your muscles do what they do best—keep you supported all the livelong day. If you're constipated, all the extra straining to get everything out pushes down against your pelvic floor muscles, which eventually weakens them and could lead to things like rectal prolapse and even more constipation.

stay active down there

Kegels are one of many simple exercises that can be beneficial for your pelvic floor. There are body-only exercises you can do, and also various contraptions that you can place inside your vagina to help do the work. But, as with any other muscly area of your body, different exercises work best for different humans—and aid in treating different forms of pelvic floor dysfunction. If they're done incorrectly, Kegels can actually intensify uncomfortable symptoms like vaginismus (involuntary tightening of vaginal muscles) or pain during sex. (Proper Kegel exercises focus on tightening/contracting your muscles and relaxing them.) Having a strong pelvic floor doesn't just mean literal muscular strength and the ability to contract—it also means having muscles that are elastic and able to flex and relax along with the movements of your body throughout your day. It's important to talk with a doctor about your unique symptoms, so you can get a treatment plan that's right for you.

try pelvic floor physical therapy

In the US, we seriously underestimate the benefits of pelvic floor physical therapy. It's been around officially for a few decades, but the idea that our pelvic floors require some special TLC goes way back in many cultures. Pelvic floor physical therapy could include exercises, manual therapy/massage, electrical stimulation, or vaginal dilators.

Whether you have any symptoms or not, discussing pelvic floor health with a qualified medical professional will set you up for a healthier, more comfortable life.

ASK
DR. JENN

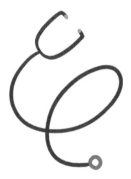

when should I start exercising my pelvic floor?

It's never too soon to be thinking about your pelvic floor, especially if you're someone who deals with chronic constipation, is overweight, or has ever given birth, regardless of delivery method (because it's likely that carrying a pregnancy, not just pushing at delivery, weakens your pelvic floor). While you may not have issues now, weak pelvic floor muscles can lead to urinary leakage, worsening constipation, and pelvic organ prolapse (where your bladder, uterus, and rectum essentially sag out of your vagina and create a bothersome bulge or even interfere with urination). It's also a good idea to talk with your provider about Kegels if you've just given birth, as both pregnancy and delivery are times of added pressure and stress on your pelvic floor muscles.

keeping your vagina happy and healthy

Dr. Jenn Conti

Chances are, vaginal health wasn't something your parents focused on during "the talk" (if you got one), and whatever sex education you had in school likely didn't mention how to evaluate vaginal discharge or itching. But despite being stigmatized AF, vaginal health is quite important.

As a gyno, I love talking about the three Ds: Douching (Don't!), Discharge, and Does it look normal? I could honestly pontificate for hours on these three topics and am absolutely guilty of having done so at dinner parties (maybe don't invite a gyno to the party next time).

Douching is an absolute no-no. What about feminine cleanses or sprays? *No.* Unscented vaginal wipes? *No.* Anything other than water? *No.* In fact, do not put anything inside your vagina for the purposes of cleaning, refreshing, or de-scenting. Your vagina is a self-cleansing ecosystem that is capable of maintaining its perfect microbiome environment. Vaginas are naturally covered in good bacteria like lactobacillus and have a baseline acidic pH that keeps everything copacetic. When you douche, you strip away your body's natural defenses and increase the likelihood of infection. And any company that tries to convince you otherwise is just trying to take your money, plain and simple!

The obvious exception to this *don't* rule is the rare occasion when life (sex, vigorous activity, other medical conditions, medications, etc.) leads to a yeast or bacterial infection and the whole pH environment down there gets thrown out of whack. In those situations, you might need antifungals or antibiotics, but douching is not the solution. Just say no!

Discharge is another common vaginal health concern, because no one ever teaches us how much is normal, what colors are normal, and which associated smells are normal. Discharge is often stigmatized and miscategorized as an automatic sign of infection, or a sign that someone is unclean. In reality, the most common reasons for changes in normal discharge are infection in the vagina, cervix, or uterus; local reactions to things like condoms, menstrual products, soaps, or detergents (or douches—don't douche!); recent antibiotics; and normal physiological changes that occur with pregnancy and menopause. It's also completely normal for everyone's discharge to be a little different. Don't compare the amount or consistency of your vaginal discharge to that of your friend. You don't have the same vagina, so you won't have the same smell or discharge.

Finally, "Does it look normal?" is another very common question I field in the gynecology office. We are so incredibly preoccupied with the way our vaginas and vulvas look, which I think is in large part due to the way society views women's bodies overall. It's not an over-reach to say that some of our ideas about what a normal vulva looks like are in part due to the way the porn industry is managed and represented. You can be sure that if all we had access to was feminist porn (which does exist, thankfully), we'd have a much broader appreciation for all variations of normal anatomy, texture, color, and size. But alas, here we are.

In the eyes of a gynecologist, "normal" is much more encompassing than you may think. As long as you don't have an infection or cancer, and as long as whatever change you've noticed isn't causing significant physical or emotional harm, it's very likely "normal."

Over the years, I have been continually shocked by the number of times people apologize for their vaginas. They apologize for not shaving or waxing before coming in, for the odor between their legs, for the blood coming out of their vaginas because they're on their periods, and for much, much more that's associated with their lady bits. My response is always the same: Don't *ever* apologize for your vagina—not to me, not to anyone. When the discharge, odor, or overall health of it is in question, there should always be an open-door policy where respectful, frank, and helpful (and sometimes hilarious) discussion ensues. If any of this isn't true, find another provider.

And never, ever douche. Ever.

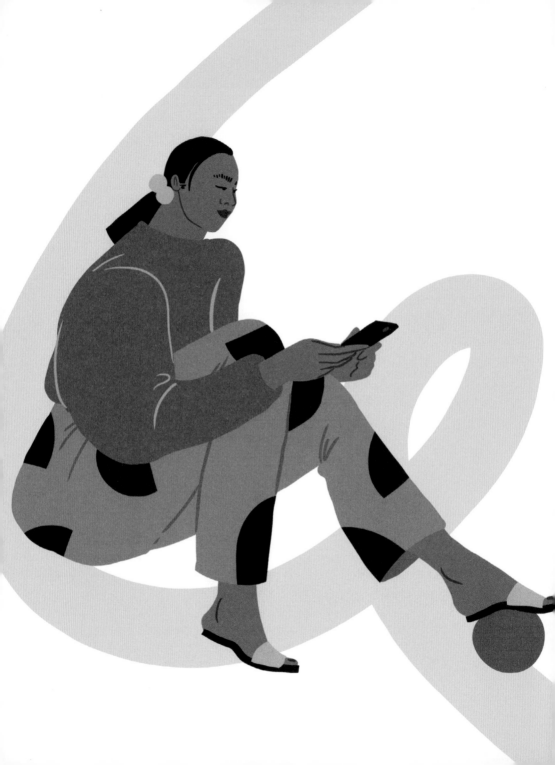

tips for developing a relationship with your gyno

Doctor visits often induce a unique kind of anxiety that can start at the moment you schedule an appointment. Now, couple those feelings of unrest with allowing someone (maybe a stranger) to examine one of your most intimate body parts while you're spread-eagled, and voilà! You've potentially entered the most awkward situation of life.

OK, stop.

Breathe.

It might seem inconceivable now, but it is possible to develop an amazing, trusting relationship with someone who has to put their fingers inside you in a nonsexual manner, despite how horrifying that sentence might seem. (Sorry.) We've put together some tips from a few of us who have figured out how to navigate the awkwardness.

Do your research. Don't just pick an ob/gyn because they're located across the street (which I've done, and it didn't work out!) or because they conveniently allowed you to book a quick appointment online. Take a few minutes to look up their ratings and reviews, and even see if they've been quoted in the news to help gauge their values. Even then, if it doesn't feel like the right fit, don't hesitate to keep looking. Just because they're the doctor doesn't mean they know your body as well as you do.

—Leesa R.

No doctor, especially one who puts stuff inside your vagina, should make you feel uncomfortable. Ever. Whether it's crappy bedside manner, judgmental advice, or the inability to validate your pain (periods can be rough, people!), remember that it's your body, that only you live in it, and that you deserve care that meets your needs—physically and emotionally. You are your best advocate, so speak up if something, anything, doesn't feel right. Don't be afraid to walk the hell outta that office if things get weird, and file a complaint with your state's Department of Health so you can help protect others from what you experienced.

—Maeve R.

If you go to a gyno once and aren't thrilled— whether it's their bed-side manner or just their general vibe—you aren't obligated to stick it out. Taking the time to find a gyno you feel good about (even if your quest lasts a decade, like mine did) is 100 percent worth it. Especially for queer folks who are tired of repeatedly explaining that they aren't on birth control because they don't have reproduc-tive sex and, no, that won't be changing anytime soon. Y'all know what I mean.

—Brianna F.

I contemplated freezing my eggs for about 4 years before I actually went through with it. Before I started seeing my current gynecologist, I didn't feel like any doctors I saw were giving me the information I needed, like actually explaining the difference between freezing an embryo or an egg. When it comes to personal decisions about your health, a doctor should never be telling you what to do with your body (yes, I have had a gyno order me to freeze my eggs when I was just asking about birth control); they should be giving you the information you need to make informed decisions for yourself.

—CJ F.

I love my gyno, but the reason I've been able to develop a comfortable relationship with her is only partially due to her down-to-earth attitude and that she's a great listener. I firmly believe that I am my body's health advocate and at each appointment, I remind myself that my doctor is working on my behalf. It's important to have the confidence to be skeptical and ask probing questions of my doctor when I want to know more. At the beginning of appointments, I explain that I like to be told what's happening throughout any exam and why, because it makes me feel taken seriously and informed about my body. I think this attitude creates the relationship I'd like to have with my gyno.

—Meredith Z.

As a gynecologist, I am privy to some of the most intimate and tender moments in a person's life, and I'm so honored to do the work that I do. People tell me things that they don't feel comfortable telling their partners, families, and closest friends. It's an incredibly intimate relationship you should feel 100 percent confident about. If you feel like your provider isn't hearing you or doesn't have your best interests in mind, try seeing someone else. As with any relationship, it's necessary to have standards you won't compromise. At the end of the day, this is about you and your health, and feeling safe and respected is an absolute must.

—Dr. Jenn

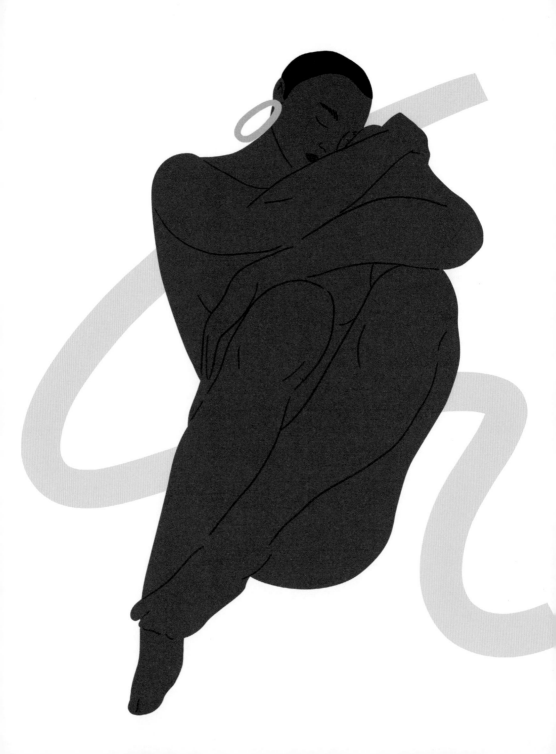

acknowledging women's pain in medical spaces

Misogyny and internalized biases about gender are still extremely powerful and embedded in our culture. Even medical spaces, which should feel safe, can perpetuate the false belief that women and femme-presenting people's experiences, emotions, and ideas are invalid—or just plain wrong.

It can be hard to recognize and confront these biases when they pop up (especially in vulnerable moments at your doctor's office), but data shows that these biases are very, very real. For one, women are less likely than men to have their pain treated appropriately when they report it to a medical professional, and, anecdotally, many women feel like doctors don't take their symptoms seriously until their condition has escalated, or has been around for years.

This is, to put it mildly, pretty damn terrible, but it's also important to understand all the ways women get dismissed in medical spaces, so we can enact real change—because there's still a lot of work to do.

women aren't weaker

As a society, we've deeply internalized the idea that women and femmes are weaker than men and masculine-presenting folks. What research actually shows is women and men communicate about their pain differently.

women are articulate about their health

Some studies have concluded that women are more forthcoming and verbal about symptoms than men, and women generally show a higher awareness of how they feel at any given moment. One of many possible explanations for this difference is that people with periods experience a monthly cycle of physical and mental symptoms, so their bodies cue them to check in more often and evaluate their health. It's also pretty likely that socialization plays a role in women being more comfortable articulating their symptoms—even though they often end up being dismissed.

women get misdiagnosed and mistreated

Even if there are major differences in how men and women experience pain, they wouldn't explain why women are often undertreated (or mistreated) when they show up at their doctor's office with legitimate health issues. One study found that doctors consistently felt female patients' symptoms were rooted in emotional issues, even when clinical tests proved otherwise. Another found that women are seven times (!) more likely than men to be misdiagnosed and discharged when they're having a heart attack—and it's all just because our understanding of medical treatment is based on the needs of—you guessed it—cisgender men.

Ultimately, everything researchers understand about gendered differences in pain—and about the experiences of women in medical spaces—is very limited. The National Institutes of Health (NIH) wasn't even legally required to include women in medical studies until 1993, so we've got some pretty serious catching up to do.

become your own health advocate

Aside from putting in the very literal blood, sweat, and tears it can take to finally find a doctor you feel you can trust (i.e., one who readily acknowledges your symptoms as valid, no matter what they might be or how you choose to share them), there are a few other key ways to make sure you're always your own best advocate in medical spaces.

do your own research

The beauty of the internet is how quickly you can learn about pretty much anything. If you've been diagnosed with a condition and offered a solution that feels wrong for you, investigate what else is out there. Pro tip: Search sites affiliated with accredited universities and institutions, and avoid getting your info from the comments in random forums. Pose questions to your doctor, and don't be afraid of questioning why they're recommending one avenue of treatment over another.

get a second opinion anytime

When it comes to major medical decisions, one person's expertise isn't always enough. It takes a little extra time and labor, but a second opinion can either reassure you or redirect your decisions about your health.

share your experiences

Whether someone else has experienced what you're going through or not, it can be good to be open about your health issues with trusted family and friends. When you isolate yourself, you can lose the feeling of support that comes from other people backing up what you're feeling, saying, or asking for.

trust your instincts

If you don't get good vibes from a doctor, get a new doctor if and when you can. If you have a procedure and something feels wrong, don't let anyone dismiss your pain or tell you everything is OK when you sense it's not. Your intuition is a powerful, valid way to assess your own health and well-being, and it's always within your rights to trust your gut.

The more you advocate for yourself in medical spaces, the more empowered you'll be to challenge biases from health professionals whenever they show up. No matter what anybody tells you, your emotional and physical well-being are always a top priority, and your understanding of your own health is the most valid.

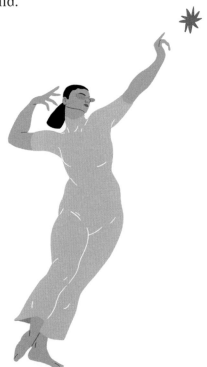

Maria Molland

on why she posts about her infertility on Instagram

I was thirty-nine years old the first time I got pregnant. It was unplanned, and I wasn't confident in my relationship at the time, but I allowed excitement to outweigh my initial hesitation.

At twenty-one weeks, I found out my baby was missing her limbs. The doctor told me it wasn't genetic; it was completely random and happens during 1 in 500,000 pregnancies. It's one of the worst kinds of lotteries a pregnant person can win. I felt an incredible amount of guilt. Even though I really wanted the baby by then, I hadn't when I first got pregnant, and thought maybe that's what caused this. Obviously, that's not how any of this works, but I couldn't stave off the thoughts. At twenty-four weeks, I had an abortion and shortly after, my boyfriend and I broke up. The procedure itself was incredibly traumatic, and I felt like the only person who had ever experienced such loss—nobody I knew was talking about these subjects. Sharing emotionally has never come easy to me, but the more I started opening up, the more I realized how wrong I was.

There were people in my life that also struggled to start their families, and I would have never known otherwise.

I knew I still wanted to be a mother despite my first experience with pregnancy, and I toyed with the idea of using a sperm donor, but I couldn't see past the pressure to have a traditional family. I married my husband 9 months after we met and soon after started IVF treatments. To be honest, I didn't think getting pregnant again would be a challenge—I had gotten pregnant by accident when I was thirty-nine, after all. I think many people, including me, spend most of their lives convinced that failing to use contraception once means getting pregnant immediately, so it's unfathomable if it's actually difficult. You never know if IVF is actually going to work, but I pumped myself full of all these unbelievably expensive drugs for 3 years.

The day I found out I was finally pregnant with my daughter was the best day of my life. I took a pregnancy test too early because I was so eager, but there was no denying that faint pink line. That December, I gave birth to Inga. Even today, every time I notice how much she has grown, or even look at a photo of her, I feel so incredibly lucky. I wouldn't change a thing about my experience, not the shots or the physical pain, but I do wish I'd known I didn't have to do it all alone. When I was getting IVF treatments, I connected with the other women at the clinic, but most of them were also going through this with their husbands at their side. I didn't have that kind of support from my husband, but even so, I realize now that I could've asked my family for help. I know that they would have shown up for me, but I didn't even ask.

When Inga was a toddler, we started talking about having another child. But then I found out my husband was being unfaithful. That was a moment of reckoning—instead of resuming IVF, I filed for divorce, free from the idea that a nuclear family was required for me to be the mother I wanted to be. Since then, I've been trying to get pregnant on my own—with a sperm donor. As part of that process, I've had two miscarriages.

This time around, I surround myself with the people I love, and I'm public about what I'm going through. I even post about it on Instagram—not for the likes, but because I know I would've felt supported during IVF, when I had the abortion, and through the scare of losing my next pregnancy, if I didn't feel like these experiences had to be secrets. Whenever I write a post about my fertility journey—even though I tend to be far more matter-of-fact than emotional—so many women reach out to share their stories in turn. I hope hearing me speak up helps them, because sharing really helps me too. Navigating infertility will never be easy—but figuring out how to shoulder these challenges together, instead of alone, will only make us stronger.

Maria is the CEO of Thinx Inc. She has over 22 years of experience in the global leadership and development of businesses at the intersection of fashion, health and wellness, sustainability, and digital media. Maria currently lives in New York City with her daughter, Inga, and their cat, Cali.

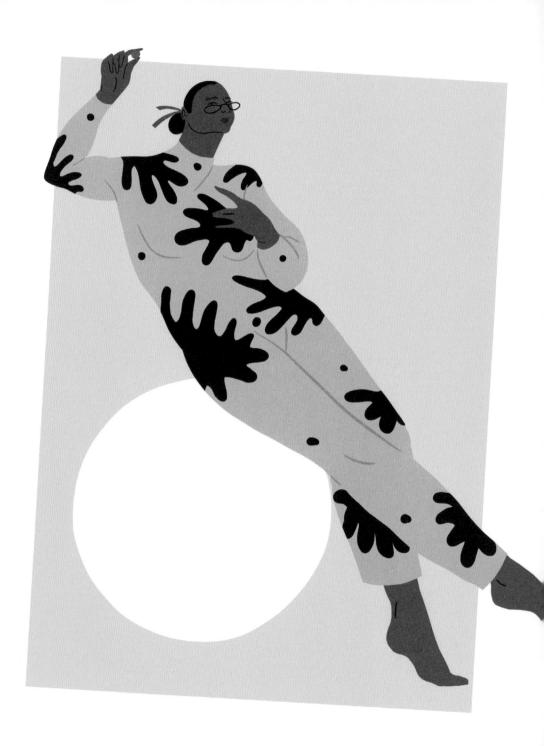

perimenopause and menopause: your period's last hurrah

For many people with periods, menopause is associated with a ton of negativity—it's a life change that can be emotional because of uncomfortable symptoms and societal stigmas around aging. Some of us have a tougher go of it than others (cue Kim Cattrall describing hot flashes as someone putting her "into a vat of boiling water") but menopause and its precursor, perimenopause, are completely natural parts of life for all people with periods.

wait, what's perimenopause?

We've heard our postmenopausal moms brag about never having to use another pad or tampon again, but perimenopause has less notoriety. In menopause (which officially starts when you haven't had a period for a full calendar year) your ovaries are no longer producing enough estrogen to release eggs, which is why menstruation starts to come to a halt. However, it takes a while for your body to get there. Perimenopause is the medical term for that slowing-down period leading up to menopause. During perimenopause, your estrogen and progesterone levels fluctuate and slowly decrease, which can wreak mild (or major) havoc on your body.

Perimenopausal symptoms typically start to show up in your forties, but perimenopause can start as early as your thirties. Some medical events, like a hysterectomy (removal of the uterus), an oophorectomy (removal of the ovaries), or certain autoimmune diseases can also trigger hormone fluctuations and cause early-onset menopause at any age. Hot flashes, mood swings, vaginal dryness, and night sweats are a few uncomfortable symptoms. Some people also gain weight, lose hair, or feel fatigued—and some carry their perimenopausal symptoms all the way into menopause and beyond.

NOTE: Once you've gone through menopause, any bleeding thereafter should be reported immediately to your gyno to rule out cancer.

what happens to your flow

Your first few periods were probably irregular, and your period's curtain call will probably be similar. If menopause is the end of a sentence, perimenopause is more like an ellipsis. It's true that some people have periods that just suddenly stop showing up, but during perimenopause, most people will experience skipped periods, irregular bleeding, spotting between periods, or a heavier or lighter flow than usual before their period officially retires. That said, when it comes to heavy bleeding, it's super important to keep your gyno in the loop. Never assume that prolonged bleeding or soaking through your period products faster than usual is something you should just have to deal with, whether you're approaching menopause or not!

a menopause survival guide

Menopause (and all the perimenopausal experiences leading up to it) can feel more than a little jarring. Talking with your doctor about methods for navigating symptoms is a great idea, but there are also a bunch of natural ways to get comfortable while change is afoot. We've suggested a few ways on the following pages.

invest in your mental health

Anxiety and depression are some of the least talked about but most common symptoms of menopause, and it's so important to recognize when it's time to reach out for help and give yourself some well-deserved TLC. Investing in mental health looks different for different people. If therapy isn't for you, trying out an exercise regimen, cutting back on caffeine, or even making a point of confiding more often in friends are a few ways to start taking care of your mental health.

commit to better sleep and relaxation practices

Many pre- and postmenopausal people have a tough time sleeping, thanks to those hormone fluctuations and night sweats. Reduced stress and anxiety are directly tied to feeling more rested and sleeping better, so trying out simple tricks like lavender essential oils, candles, and even leaving your phone in another room when you sleep can all help foster some calming vibes before bed.

create your own climate control

Hot flashes aren't a given for everybody, but they're a big reason why this time in a person's life gets such a bad rap. That said, there are a bunch of ways to keep cool year-round, and sometimes simple remedies are best. Whether it's a cup of ice or a good old-fashioned wet rag in the freezer, you just need to find the solution that's best for your body.

pay attention to your body

Sometimes undetected conditions—like nutritional deficiencies or thyroid problems—can actually intensify menopause symptoms. Plus, during and after menopause, you're at increased risk for conditions like osteoporosis, bladder leaks, and cardiovascular disease. It's important to stay in tune with your body as a whole, in addition to the new changes and symptoms demanding your attention.

allow yourself to keep growing

If our collective experiences in middle school were any indication, a hormonal shift is a huge opportunity for growth and change. In the words of Oprah, "So many women I've talked to see menopause as an ending. But I've discovered this is your moment to reinvent yourself after years of focusing on the needs of everyone else." Because menopause is a timestamp in your life, it's also an opportunity to reevaluate, recalibrate, and redirect anything that doesn't feel perfectly suited to *you*.

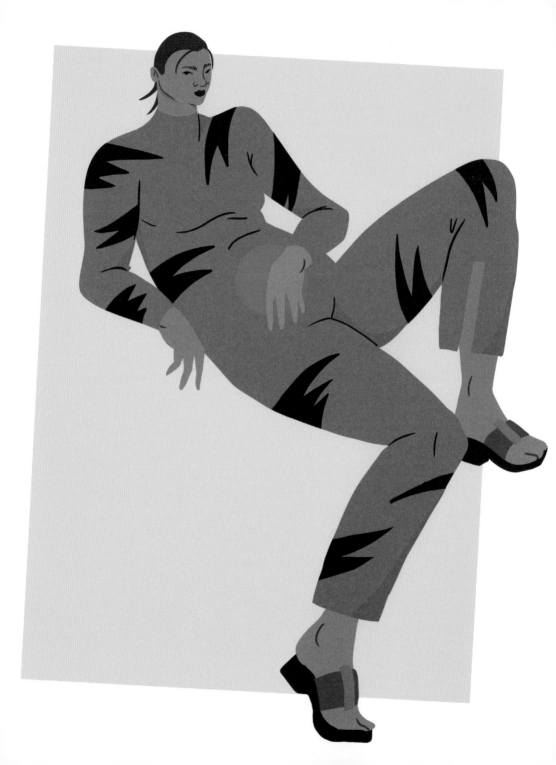

fertility
fact or fiction?

Conversations about fertility are often shrouded in secrecy. And when those conversations do happen, they're often filled with incorrect assumptions or colored by superstitions. This aversion to talking frankly about how people do (or don't) get pregnant has made it pretty difficult to separate the facts from the fiction. Let's set the story straight about a few persistent myths.

birth control causes infertility: fiction

A common misconception is that if you've been taking a hormonal birth control like the pill for an extended period of time, it affects your ability to conceive. This is not the case. However, it could take up to a couple months for ovulation to resume after stopping birth control, which could explain the worry. Basically, your body might need some extra time to figure out how to get back to running your menstrual cycle naturally.

you're born with all of your eggs: fact

Most people with vaginas are born with 1 to 2 million eggs, and instead of producing more as you age, you just start losing them at a pretty drastic rate. By the time puberty and first periods start, that number is usually down to about 350,000 to 400,000 eggs. In contrast, sperm is produced every 70 days.

if you conceive naturally once, it'll be easy to do it again: fiction

People with ovaries don't have consistent fertility throughout life, because as you age, the number and quality of eggs decreases. Talk to your doctor if you do struggle to conceive again; they'll be able to help you figure out the best course of action for you and your family.

it's impossible to conceive naturally after a certain age: fiction

While the probability of getting pregnant does lessen as you age, as long as you aren't past menopause (roughly 48 to 55 years old), pregnancy could happen if you're having unprotected sex. So yup, it's still important to use contraception if you'd like to avoid procreating and still worth talking to your doctor about your options if you do want to have a child. There are more risks associated with pregnancy when you're over forty, but that's why keeping a trusted gyno in the loop is key.

breastfeeding is birth control: fiction

People who are breastfeeding can definitely get pregnant. Tell all your friends! This myth is probably so commonly perpetuated because exclusively breastfeeding a baby (around the clock, with no formula) can delay the return of menstruation and ovulation. If you wait until you have a period before worrying about getting on birth control, remember that ovulation occurs two weeks before. If you are breastfeeding your baby, your options for hormonal birth control will also be limited for the first few weeks after you give birth. It can be easy to feel overwhelmed by everything that comes with taking care of a new baby, so try to nail down a plan for contraception with your doctor before you take your little bundle of joy home. Even if resuming a sex life after you give birth is the last thing you care about at that moment, getting a plan in place will be one thing you won't have to worry about later.

only women can be infertile: fiction

Contrary to what goes on in *A Handmaid's Tale* (and what far too many people IRL actually believe) fertility struggles have a variety of causes and include the fertility of the person who's supposed to be providing the sperm. Sperm production can be affected by diet, stress, how much sleep someone gets, and a whole bunch of things that have nothing to do with a vagina. If you and your partner are struggling to conceive, it's important that both of you speak to your doctor, and don't let weird, patriarchal ideas affect what's probably already an emotional time in your relationship.

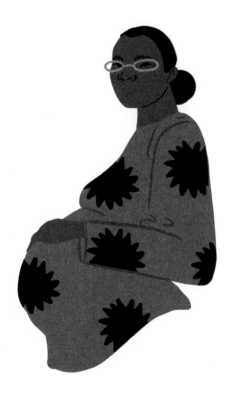

Latham Thomas

on why we need to step up for black mothers—
and where we can start

Two months after the blissful birth of my son, the birth center where I delivered him was shut down because it couldn't afford the skyrocketing insurance premiums. Elizabeth Seton Childbearing Center had been the only freestanding birth center in New York City, and a pillar of excellence in the birth community, so I began advocating for a replacement. That was when I started to track the war on women's rights to give birth the way they desire. I found myself surrounded by white women who envisioned a future of birth for themselves,

but I didn't see anyone who looked like me standing up for women of color, even though I knew birth mattered deeply to Black women.

In 2017 ProPublica issued the groundbreaking report "Nothing Protects Black Women from Dying in Pregnancy and Childbirth: Not education. Not income. Not even being an expert on racial disparities in health care." The following year, the *New York Times* ran "Why America's Black Mothers and Babies Are in a Life-or-Death Crisis: The answer to the disparity in death rates has everything to do with the lived experience of being a Black woman in America." Black women finally had the nation's attention. Our stories were finally being told by the mainstream media.

The lives of Black women are not prioritized by our current medical model. We know that more women in America are dying of pregnancy-related complications than in any other developed country—and only in the United States has the rate of maternal deaths actually risen. There are no federally mandated standard hospital protocols for dealing with potentially fatal complications, so treatable complications become lethal. According to the ProPublica report, only 6 percent of block grants for "maternal and child health" actually go to the health of mothers. Some doctors entering the growing specialty of maternal-fetal medicine are able to complete that training without ever spending time in a labor and delivery unit. And the complex history of this country renders women of color especially vulnerable—we need to address the implicit

bias in clinical settings that is steeped in white supremacy. If we focus our attention on improving maternal health outcomes for Black women, everyone's birth outcomes will improve.

I recently spoke to a thirty-seven-year-old woman named Jasmine, who has been thinking a lot about having a baby. She's Black, educated, and just beginning to explore her options. At a checkup with her midwife, it became clear that media reports about Black maternal health birth outcomes were giving her anxiety. Jasmine broke down crying. She wasn't even aware that she was carrying so much anxiety about the uncertainty of safety, and she realized that she was paralyzed with fear by the thought of pregnancy.

When it comes to the news cycle, we have to remember to take back how our stories are being told. These are lives, not just numbers and data points. It's critical to honor those whose lives have been lost, but we have to counter the challenging, emotionally draining stories with ones of triumph too. Awareness is important, but there comes a time when too much exposure to a subject can incapacitate you, and we don't want to invite a narrative for Black families that says it's not safe to have a baby, so they shouldn't even try. Instead, we must affirm and empower ourselves and each other with information, support, and advocacy tools for survival.

We need to examine the weathering toll all of this is taking on Black bodies and how it can render us vulnerable before we even get pregnant. We need to create our provider dream teams of doctors, midwives, doulas, nutritionists, and mental health practitioners who will serve on the front lines and protect the safety and sanctity of birth. We need community support to help us achieve the seemingly insurmountable task of improving our maternal and neonatal health outcomes. Access to this work and support isn't a luxury—it's a necessity.

Latham is a celebrity wellness/lifestyle maven and birth doula. Named one of Oprah Winfrey's SuperSoul 100, Latham is the founder of Mama Glow, New York's premiere maternity lifestyle brand and women's center, with hubs in Brooklyn, Paris, and LA. Mama Glow offers full-spectrum doula support along the childbearing continuum and is home to the fastest-growing doula education program in the US. With clients including Alicia Keys, DJ Khaled, Rebecca Minkoff, and more, Latham is leading a revolution in radical self-care.

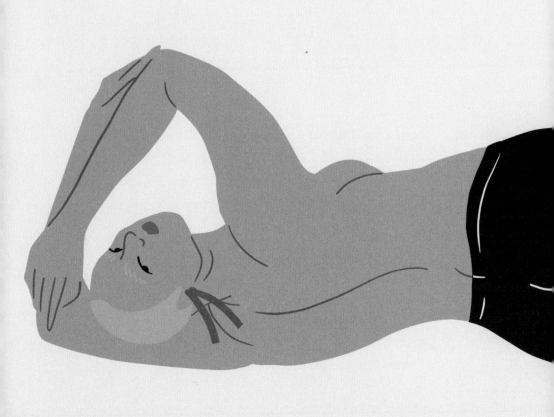

CHAPTER 3

sex & contraception

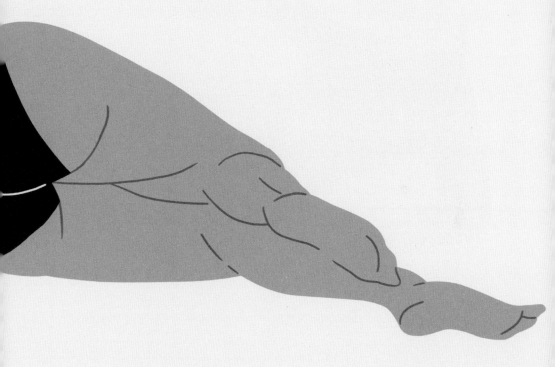

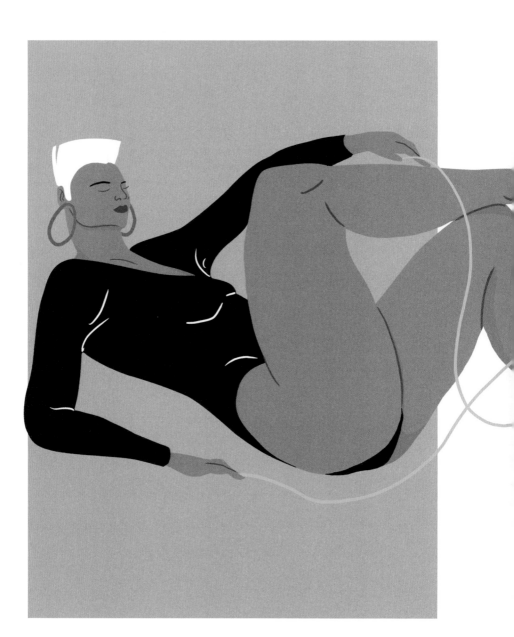

exploring
your sexuality

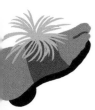

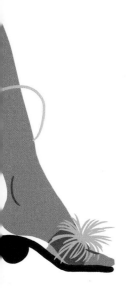

You've heard the story: Boy meets girl, yadda yadda yadda, and then they live happily ever after! In reality, girl may not like boy (or boys in general), or she may wake up one day with a craving for a little something else—at the very least she certainly deserves a voice in her own narrative. Often, sexual exploration is portrayed in the media as some steamy run-in at a bar bathroom, or the perversions of an isolated sect, but the reality is that curiosity and open-mindedness toward your own desires can be a lifelong journey. No one can tell you what feels good for you like you can, and exploring and discovering your own passions, desires, kinks, turn-ons, and sexual identity is an important part of self-actualization and a cornerstone of healthy relationships.

hearts not parts

Many people's first sexual act is a fantasy or masturbation, but eventually other people might get involved in their sexual experiences. As soon as sex hormones start developing, adolescents can become curious about their own sex organs as well as the sex organs and sexuality of others. And sometimes that just never stops!

Most of us learned in sex ed class that sex is when a penis is inserted into a vagina, but that definition is far from comprehensive. Sex can be any form of sexual gratification, whether or not that includes penetration or even a penis and a vagina. Despite heterosexuality dominating social, cultural, and political domains for millennia, studies show that fewer and fewer people identify as "completely heterosexual."

Sexual orientation can develop and emerge over time, and this is rarely a linear process. For far too many people who don't fit the heteronormative paradigm, self-actualization may not feel like a safe option, and it's important to recognize that cultural, political, and religious contexts may make some sexual exploration more difficult to pursue or, in some places, even illegal. Because of this, all people, regardless of their sexuality or sexual preferences, should encourage freedom of sexual expression for everyone.

what gets you going?

Sexual pleasure can come from a wide range of activities and actions. Some people might like a little dirty talk, others might be into filming their escapades (disable iCloud now). We aren't here to tell you what gets you off, but if you're feeling a little frisky and want some places to start, here are some options to explore:

- the wide world of kinks and fetishes
- sex toys
- role play
- pornography
- orgies or play parties
- BDSM
- your imagination!

It's important to listen to your body and mind when you feel a pull to these activities. Sexual expression between two consenting adults (or one sexy solo) can be healthy. However, if you find that you're uncomfortable with some of your desires or their origins, or if there are certain practices that start to overwhelm your life, it's worth taking a look at what's driving you. Speaking up about your feelings to your partner, trusted friends, or even a professional about the way you're feeling—being honest while you're exploring—is key.

how to get started

The beginning of any sexual encounter should be a conversation with yourself. What are you interested in feeling or exploring, and where do you want to draw the line? This can be a quick check-in the moment the possibility of any given experience arises. Some of the best experiences can be spontaneous, but you owe it to yourself to come back to reality for a hot sec with a quick "Am I OK with this? y/n/m."

After you've thought about what you want to get out of a physical or emotional connection, this might be something to bring up with someone you're interested in sharing the moment with. Start by having a conversation with your partner(s) about opening up a new type of connection. Be mindful and respectful, though; the person you know who has a certain sexual practice does not exist to serve your curiosity or fantasy. They have their own wants, needs, and preferences. Just because you know a sub doesn't mean they want to be *your* sub.

what's safe?

Broadly speaking, the rules of engagement are that sexual exploration should be mutually agreed upon: not coerced; not causing extreme anger, shame, fear, or anxiety; and (and we can't stress this enough) *safe*. By safe, we mean protecting your physical and emotional safety first and foremost. For any and all sexual activity involving others, you must give (and seek) specific, enthusiastic, and informed consent, even if you're in a situation where activity might seem inevitable or asked for.

Unfortunately, most of us weren't taught in health class how to have safe sex if you're not heterosexual, or what consent means in a BDSM relationship. If you're unsure about how to stay safe in a new situation or community, you should start by doing your research. However, general rules of thumb are: penises should wear condoms, BDSM scenes should have a safe word, and even if you're into gags, make sure you always have a clear line of communication available. If you find yourself in a position where you feel any of these rules are potentially not being followed, or something just doesn't feel right, remove yourself from the situation. And if you find yourself struggling to process any encounter, don't be afraid to seek help! Not to sound like a broken record, but there should be no shame in discussing uncomfortable sexual encounters.

where's the line?

The boundaries of what is an emotionally safe interaction are defined differently for everyone. Most partnerships leave space for individuals to communicate about what experimentation is permitted within the relationship. Your partner(s) and you may want to have a formal conversation defining what is permissible exploration and what behavior could be detrimental to your arrangement. Which sexual acts, online interactions, conversations, topics, and physical touches feel hurtful to you if your partner(s) engage in them? Is it OK to like photos of other people? Is talking about your sexual desires with someone outside the relationship OK? Coming up with these ground rules early in a relationship can help avoid some hurts later when @yourboo likes all of @notyourboo's posts. For many of us, emotional cheating is cheating too.

Sexual exploration can be a tool for self-discovery and reaching new levels of passion and excitement with others. As with most things in life, be safe and you'll have fun.

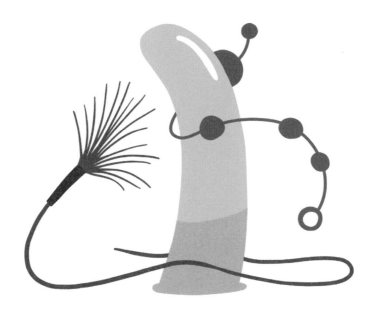

unveiling the mysteries of orgasms

Dr. Jenn Conti

If there's one thing we in the medical field know about orgasms, it's that we don't know enough. Studying female sexual health has historically been deemed taboo, and is consequently underrepresented in medical school education, research, and even public discussion. Luckily, orgasms happen whether you understand them or not, so it's worth breaking down all the details as clearly as possible, and then talking about why we don't know enough about this part of women's health. After all, everyone deserves to experience orgasms, and often.

In French literature, there is a euphemism referring to an orgasm: *la petite mort* (the little death)—as the British poet, Percy Shelley, so famously described, "No life can equal such a death." So, what is an orgasm and why does it exist? Medically, it's the rapid, pleasurable release of neuromuscular tensions at a point in the sexual response cycle that results in genital muscle spasms and euphoria (from feel-good brain chemicals). Culturally, it's so much more.

Orgasming—having the Big O, climaxing, getting off, and however else you've heard it described—is almost synonymous with sex, but unfortunately not assured for all people with vaginas.

In a 2010 study conducted in the United States, researchers found that about 40 percent of US women reported problems attaining orgasm. The numbers are similar for women across other countries studied, including the United Kingdom, Mexico, and Australia. Queer women are not well represented in this data, but separate, smaller studies estimate similar rates as well. The causes of this are multifactorial and also—you guessed it—not as well understood as they should be, but often include psychosocial and cultural factors, as well as issues from medical conditions or medications.

One explanation for this disparity between the number of women having sex and those having orgasms is the pervasive sex industry in our society that suggests sex for women looks a certain way (which isn't realistic to start with), and anything that deviates from that is wrong or abnormal. Porn, mainstream television, movies, and marketing campaigns traditionally focus on sexual pleasure through a male lens. Only recently have innovators in these respective industries started changing the narrative with more feminist and inclusive tones.

Some groundbreaking examples of this include subscription audio stories and apps (Dipsea, Rosy) that focus on the emotional and psychosocial buildup that is often crucial for the female sexual response cycle, and mostly missing from mainstream porn and mass media. There are even subscription services like

Slutbot that coach you on how to improve your sexting skills by practicing talking dirty in safe spaces. The central theme of these services is that they're normalizing nonheterosexual, non-male-centric sexual pleasure, and teaching people that bulldozing toward an orgasm doesn't work for many people with vaginas. You shouldn't be surprised to hear that the mainstream porn industry has greatly misrepresented orgasms.

For example, while orgasms vary wildly in terms of type, intensity, and length, many people need some degree of clitoral stimulation to actually feel an orgasm. This can happen through direct contact with the clitoris or even indirect contact via nearby vaginal penetration.

The alleged "G-spot," named after German gynecologist Ernst Gräfenberg, is the so-called sweet spot in the vagina that, when stimulated, leads to strong sexual arousal and orgasm. Whether or not it actually exists is up for debate, as its exact location and structure have never been reliably identified. Many sexology experts believe it is instead likely an extension of the clitoris. The problem with sensationalizing the existence of the G-spot is that it insinuates that people who don't get pleasure via vaginal stimulation alone must have something wrong with them, which is not true at all.

There is no singular, correct way to achieve sexual pleasure, and no set standards for what good sex looks like, so long as you're happy and healthy in your endeavors. Our understanding of sexual health is evolving and so is our appreciation for more open-minded narratives.

ASK DR. JENN

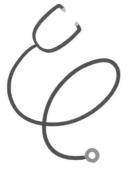

I can't orgasm, no matter how hard I try. Help!

Believe it or not, many people with vaginas can't orgasm through penetration alone and require some sort of clitoral stimulation to get the job done. If, try as you might, you still can't orgasm, even with dedicated clitoris time, there are a plethora of amazing resources out there to check out, like OMGyes (an online, interactive tutorial on pleasure, to use with or without a partner) and Juicebox (a remarkably affordable online sexual health counseling service that can help with targeted goals like achieving orgasm).

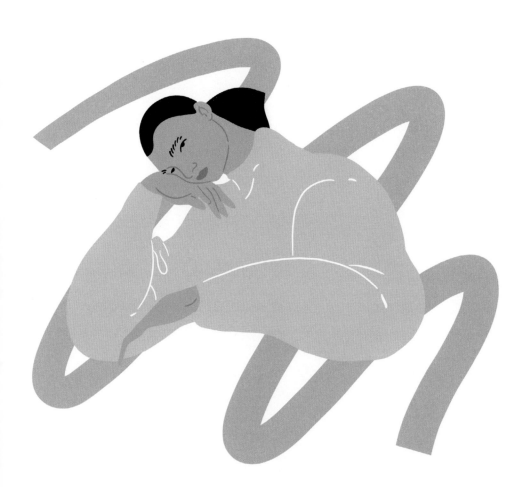

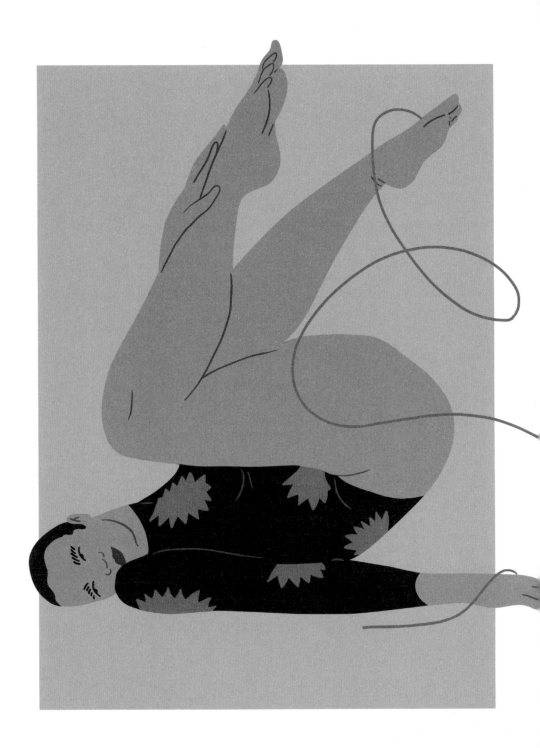

the health benefits of masturbation

Even though we have made tremendous strides toward a more sex-positive world, masturbation is still a taboo that many associate with outdated stereotypes and shame. While it can be an uncomfortable topic for some, we hope to continue pushing forward a more flattering narrative surrounding self-pleasure through education. Solo-sex desires are completely natural; a large percentage of people masturbate (like, literally everyone), so you are not alone! Masturbation is enjoyable, satisfying, and the ultimate act of self-care, plus there are pretty valuable health benefits that come along with taking some sexy *you* time. We've put together a list of a few.

orgasms produce happy chemicals

Post-orgasm, your body releases endorphins, dopamine, oxytocin, and vasopressin—brain chemicals that have a similar makeup to morphine, and operate to make you feel good, regulate your mood, and naturally relieve pain. These happy chemicals also lower your cortisol levels (cortisol causes inflammation, stress, and other unwanted issues).

help you get to know *you*

Sexuality is difficult to define and completely different for each of us. There isn't some written manuscript that we can all refer to for step-by-step instructions. Getting to know exactly what you like in the bedroom isn't necessarily straightforward; it often takes some trial and error to discover your preferences and define your boundaries. But the enormous payoff is that masturbation can boost your self-image and improve your self-esteem. Improving self-image and self-esteem through solo play is the perfect way to learn your sexual preferences and desires. And if you choose to engage with a partner, that solo time can equip you to request a healthier, more positive pleasure playground.

alleviate PMS symptoms

Masturbating while you're on your period can actually ease cramps. During orgasm, contractions help to expel blood and tissue from the uterine cavity. (Sexy!) Also, those happy endorphins not only give your mood a boost but also relieve pain, which is good news for those who experience migraines and cluster headaches.

get those ZZZZZs

Getting some quality hours of sleep is essential for conquering the day, and DIY sex comes through for the win again! Masturbating increases relaxation (well, after orgasm), reduces cortisol hormone levels, and is a great, nonaddictive way to increase your quality of sleep. The combination of oxytocin and additional hormones released during masturbation is nature's sedative. More and better sleep equals a stronger immune system and more energy during the day.

Polly Rodriguez

on the feminist history of the vibrator

At twenty-one years old, I found myself on the tan, cold plastic of an oncologist's examining chair in St. Louis, Missouri, as my doctor told me that radiation to shrink the tumor in my colon would result in lifelong infertility. A few weeks later, I googled my symptoms when my hot flashes grew almost unbearable, and discovered that I was also going through menopause.

A friend who was a nurse graciously explained that menopause (of which I knew next to nothing) would result in a dip in libido and vaginal dryness.

Translation: If I wanted to continue enjoying sex, I should probably invest in a vibrator and some lubricant, which is how I ended up at the Hustler Hollywood next to the St. Louis airport, staring at a mannequin in a crotchless onesie. I felt like a sexual deviant. What I didn't know was 1 in 3 women in the United States regularly use a vibrator. Many women need clitoral stimulation (which rarely occurs during penetrative sex) in order to climax. In fact, 40 percent of women report chronic difficulty reaching orgasm, compared with less than 7 percent of men. But my gym teacher didn't even utter the word "clitoris" in my seventh-grade sex ed class, so how could I have known any of this?

As I stood under the harsh fluorescent lights of that store, tugging on the brim of my baseball cap to conceal as much of my face as possible, I couldn't help but wonder why buying a vibrator felt like an undercover sting operation. Why were vibrators treated like contraband? How did we get here?

As it turns out, the vibrator has quite a history. When Joseph Mortimer Granville invented the electric vibrator in the late 1880s, the technology was considered revolutionary. Ads for vibrators could be found in a Sears Roebuck catalog, claiming to cure everything from headaches to constipation. Vibrators were considered a household staple, but not for long.

Less than a year after film was invented in 1880, pornography made its debut. By the 1920s, vibrators were often featured in pornographic content. It became widely known they were being used for—*gasp*—the sexual pleasure of women, and thus they became a symbol of perversion. They were quickly plucked from mainstream shopping catalogs and relegated to the shadows. As a result, in the decades that followed, vibrators were considered lewd products that could only be bought alongside porno magazines at strip malls and truck stops across America.

Vibrators didn't resurface into the cultural zeitgeist until the 1970s. Feminist icon Betty Dodson spoke out about the crucial role masturbation should play in the women's liberation movement. She hosted masturbation workshops in her New York City loft, encouraging women to use Hitachi Magic Wands to reach orgasm. And Betty was only the beginning.

In 1974, Dell Williams opened Eve's Garden, the first woman-owned and -operated sex toy business in the United States. Joani Blank opened Good Vibrations in 1977, which grew into nine retail locations. Not only did these sex-positive shops provide a welcoming space to buy vibrators, they also offered safe spaces for women to learn about their bodies. Shops like Babeland hosted small educational seminars where anyone could come and learn about sexual interests without judgment or shame.

Yet still, unlike erectile dysfunction drugs and condom brands, vibrator companies are considered "morally offensive" by most financial institutions and advertising platforms. They're banned from advertising on Facebook, Instagram, Pinterest, Twitter, Snapchat, Reddit, YouTube, the subway, television, radio, and the list goes on. Everything from opening a bank account to getting health insurance for your employees becomes a massive hurdle when you're a sex tech company founder (which I happen to be).

Despite these deeply rooted, systemic institutional barriers, sex tech continues to forge ahead, creating innovative products, platforms, and experiences for sexual health and wellness. We continue to fight for the right to make decisions for our bodies, be it access to reproductive healthcare or pleasure and vibrators.

I'm hopeful the next generation won't have to dress up in a trench coat and baseball cap in order to buy their first vibrator. We shouldn't be ashamed of the tools we use to help us explore and enjoy our bodies.

Polly is the CEO and cofounder of Unbound, a rebellious sexual wellness company. Polly and Sarah Jayne started Unbound with the goal of taking vibrators, lubricants, and sexual accessories mainstream through elevated design, body-safe materials, and accessible pricing. Today, the company has been hailed by the *New York Times* as the "ideological center of the tech-savvy, female-led women's sexuality movement" with over fifty products created by a team of ten women in New York City.

a contraception and STI prevention cheat sheet

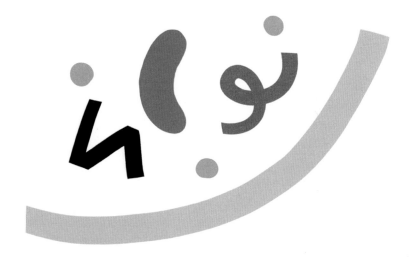

We all know in theory that practicing safe sex is essential, but there are a whole lot of intimidating choices to make when it comes to contraception, whether that's choosing hormones, committing to a daily contraceptive, or signing up for a minor procedure. Let's walk through the more popular options for contraception. If you're interested in learning more about using one of them, follow up with your gyno!

CONDOMS

85 percent effective*

Hormonal birth control can prevent pregnancy, but condoms are still necessary to protect you from STIs. Used alone, condoms are 98 percent effective in preventing pregnancy when used perfectly. Using a condom incorrectly (or a condom breaking) happens more frequently than you might think—the typical failure rate is actually 13 percent. Make sure to purchase the correct size, never reuse a condom, and opt for water or silicone-based lubes (any other products mess with latex).

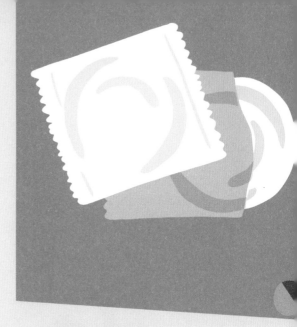

INTERNAL CONDOMS

79 percent effective

Chances are, you saw an internal or "female" condom unwrapped in a sex ed class, and then never saw one again. Like their male condom counterparts, internal condoms can protect from STIs, but there is a bit of a learning curve when it comes to insertion. They're a good alternative for people who are allergic to latex, and can be inserted up to 8 hours before intercourse.

THE PILL

91 percent effective

There are so many different types that finding a daily contraceptive pill that works with your body can feel like playing a game of Russian roulette. Side effects aside, the pill is still a very popular and accessible option. Tracking the changes to your body when you start any new medication will give you information to evaluate whether to stick with it.

THE PATCH
91 percent effective
Uses the same hormones as the combined pill (estrogen and progestin), but you only have to worry about it once a week. You place the patch like a sticker on one of the approved parts of your body, and that's it!

THE IMPLANT
99 percent effective
A small plastic rod that's inserted into your upper arm and prevents pregnancy for 3 years by releasing the hormone progestin. And while the FDA has approved its use for 3 years, newer research shows it is effective for up to 5 years!

IUD
99 percent effective
An intrauterine device (IUD) is a T-shaped piece of plastic inserted into your uterus. Hormonal IUDs release progestin, while the hormone-free option is made of copper, which is toxic to sperm. IUDs are effective from 3 to 12 years (depending on the model) and can be removed at any time.

THE SHOT
94 percent effective
Between taking a pill every day and the commitment of an IUD or implant lies the Depo-Provera shot, which is progestin-based and only requires a quarterly visit to your doctor or clinic.

THE RING
91 percent effective
NuvaRing is a small, flexible ring placed inside your vagina that you replace monthly (including a week off for a period). It releases estrogen and progestin.

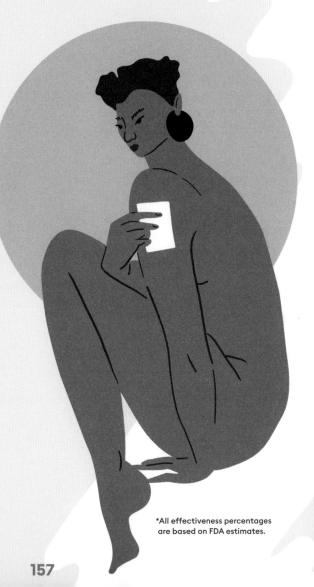

*All effectiveness percentages are based on FDA estimates.

FERTILITY AWARENESS

Also called "natural family planning" or the "rhythm method," fertility awareness involves carefully tracking your menstrual cycle (and most importantly, ovulation), so you know exactly when your fertile days will be. People use fertility awareness either to avoid pregnancy or to conceive. A few methods for doing so are keeping a physical calendar to chart your cycle, monitoring your basal body temperature (temperature when resting, which should be higher when you ovulate), and observing your cervical mucus (its consistency changes during your cycle). Still, due to the possibility of large margins of error, fertility awareness isn't an ideal singular method to avoid pregnancy.

DIAPHRAGMS

88 percent effective

A flexible, shallow saucer inserted into your vagina that covers your cervix. To effectively avoid pregnancy, it must be used every time you have sex, and ideally used in conjunction with spermicide, a chemical that kills sperm. Even when used perfectly, diaphragms are 88 percent effective (and the complicated insertion process leaves a lot of room for error).

DENTAL DAMS

Used for oral sex, dental dams are thin pieces of latex that prevent direct mouth-to-genital contact and protect you from STIs.

NOTE: It's important to practice all kinds of safe sex with new partners, including requesting current test results if you're interested in engaging in unprotected sex.

what we wish we had known about hormonal birth control

For many of us, a relationship with hormonal birth control is just like any other. There are brief flings with pill packs that make us way too sad, long-term codependency with that cute little IUD, a torrid love triangle between—OK, you get the picture. If the opportunity arose, most of us would love to warn our young, naïve selves that there's a birth control out there that will break your heart (or at the very least, give you some crazy severe acne). Here are some lessons a few of our friends wish they could tell their younger selves.

It's not for everyone, but it might be for you! There can be a lot of shame and misinformation about birth control—everyone seems to have an opinion. Don't listen to the fearmongers. Only a supportive gynecologist you feel comfortable with can come up with the right plan. Don't ignore any side effects, however minor or vain they might seem (yes, my birth control gives me a hyperpigmentation mustache), keep track of everything, and come prepared for that important conversation with your doctor.

—Hilary F. G.

I wish I knew how the pill actually worked when I started taking it almost 10 years ago. When I was sixteen, it was a magical way to regulate my heavy period and reduce accompanying symptoms. But when I started having sex, I never learned how it protected me from getting pregnant—that the hormones the pill released prevented me from experiencing the dip in hormones that would naturally occur on a monthly basis and cause me to ovulate. That after 7 days of taking the pill (at the same time each day), back-up birth control was not required. It took a college biology class for me to learn this, and I was struck by the fact that no healthcare professional had ever explained this to me. It felt really empowering to know the science behind the pill.

—Meredith Z.

I was not informed just how drastic the depression side effects could be for hormonal birth control. I was experiencing very dark thoughts 2 months in and was simply told I had to tough it out for another month.

—Morgan R.

I wish I felt more validated using birth control as a period management tool when I was a teenager. My early periods were really heavy, like, bleeding-through-a-super-tampon-every-1½-hours heavy. My mom and doctor were cool about me going on birth control to manage it, but I always felt like I had to justify my need to friends and the world at large. —Sam P.

It definitely would have helped if I had been given more information about how to take the pill properly. Like what time of day was best, whether or not that should be the same time every day, what to do if I wanted to stop taking it, or if there were side effects I was supposed to be aware of that weren't normal. —Denise C.

Going off the pill can throw your cycle out of whack! When I was ready to get pregnant, I went off the pill after 10-plus years of baby-free hormonal regulation. I expected to be with child before dinner. What really happened was I didn't have a period for 6 months, and then it took another 6 months until I had a monthly flow. This didn't keep me from getting pregnant, but it did make it harder to understand when I was ovulating. It took longer than expected, but now I have a super cute baby girl and the knowledge that when it's time for kiddo #2, I should say goodbye to the pill way sooner than I previously thought.

—Maeve R.

Especially growing up as an athlete, doctors were constantly trying to prescribe me birth control to solve almost every problem I came to them with. I'm still not on birth control, and I wish that someone had assured me that I didn't need to be, despite so much pressure to do so (especially since having sex definitely doesn't always mean having sex with someone who can get you pregnant).

—Carolyn K.

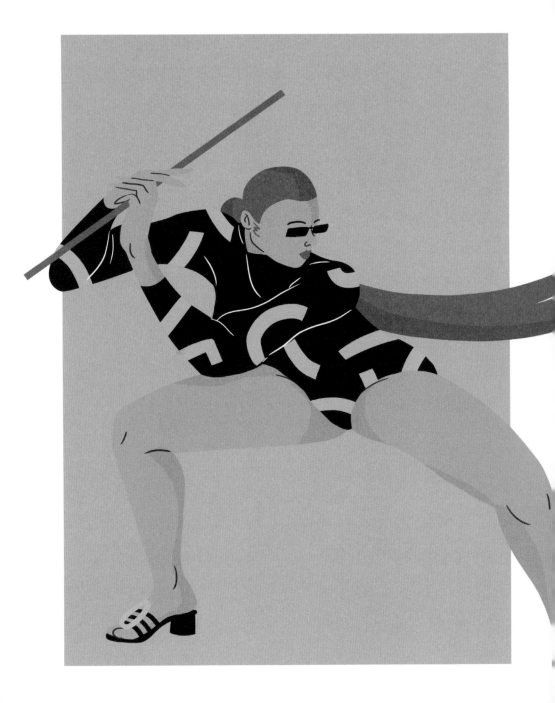

the freak-out-free guide to STIs

There's probably nothing that feels less sexy than talking about sexually transmitted diseases and infections with a current or potential partner. But starting conversations is an important piece of practicing safe sex—the more you know about that scary stuff, the more comfortable and equipped you'll be to protect your and your partners' health.

The acronyms STI (sexually transmitted infection) and STD (sexually transmitted disease) can get confusing, but STI is gaining traction as a more inclusive term, because it covers both disease and viral infections. Some of the most common infections (like gonorrhea or chlamydia) may not have signs or symptoms, and it's not until they progress that they could become a "disease."

who's actually at risk?

Many people think it's only important to get tested for STIs if you're sexually active with more than one partner. The truth is that some STIs can lurk in the body for months or years before any physical symptoms show up, so even someone in a long-term, mutually monogamous relationship can test positive for an STI that they might've thought they didn't have a few years back. Per the Centers for Disease Control and Prevention (CDC), everyone who is sexually active under the age of twenty-five should be tested for chlamydia and gonorrhea every year, and then again when they engage with new partners. The CDC also recommends everyone get tested for HIV at least once in their lifetime, and that people who have other risk factors get tested at least once a year. Don't ever be ashamed or embarrassed about getting tested; your personal information is confidential, and you can even explore anonymous testing if that's a concern. It's so important to look out for number one (you).

When it comes to sexual health, knowledge is definitely power, so here's a primer about symptoms and treatment of some of the most common STIs.

chlamydia

Like many other STIs, chlamydia can come as a surprise—most people don't experience symptoms in the
early stages (if at all), and when symptoms do show
up, you might just think you're having the worst infection of your life. But if you notice abdominal pain, pain
during sex, and frequent or painful peeing, it's time
to visit your doctor. A simple urine test will reveal if
chlamydia is the cause, and if it is, your doctor will send
you home with antibiotics for you and your partner(s).
Partner therapy is something most major medical
bodies recommend, otherwise people tend to just pass
the infection back and forth.

HPV

HPV, or human papillomavirus, is pretty much the
common cold of STIs. Most people you know will have
it at some point or another, and a lot of people fight off
the virus before it ever shows up on a test. That said,
it's important for people with vaginas to get tested for
HPV every 1 to 3 years, because it can eventually lead to
certain types of cancer. Since there are so many different strains of the virus, testing is the only reliable way
to know if you're in the clear or not, so make sure you
don't skip your pap smears (as tempting as that may
be). If you do test positive, your doctor can work with
you to monitor the virus and make sure it clears up.
You can also ask whether you're eligible for the HPV
vaccine, which helps protect against some of the most
common strains.

gonorrhea

Gonorrhea can be present without symptoms and go unnoticed in many people (just like chlamydia), but can lead to infertility in both men and women. Its symptoms—which include green or yellow discharge, a burning sensation while peeing, and spotting between periods—should signal an immediate doctor visit. If you test positive, they'll send you home with antibiotics, and off you'll go to heal and get back to having better, safer sex.

herpes

It's pretty safe to say that herpes is the most stigmatized STI out there. It's incurable, it's highly contagious, and more than 1 in 6 people in the US have it. Plus, most people who have it will never even know (and yes, it is possible to infect someone else when you have no symptoms, although it's less common). People who do have visible symptoms (i.e., an outbreak of genital warts, or cold sores on or around your mouth) are saddled with the burden of having to explain to potential sexual partners that it's completely possible to have safe, enjoyable sex with a partner who has herpes.

It can take weeks, months, and even years for a visible outbreak to pop up. If you notice a blister (or you can't tell if it's just an ingrown hair), schedule a checkup with your doctor, who can help you get to the bottom of what's going on. If you do have herpes, there are medications that can help manage uncomfortable outbreaks, and your doctor can educate you on how to have safe sex with your current and future partners.

Using protection, getting tested regularly, and visiting your doctor when you have a question or concern are the three simplest ways to take control of your sexual health. The bottom line is that the more open and educated you are, the better you can protect your health, and the health of current and future partners.

ASK DR. JENN

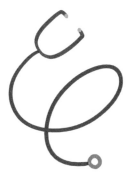

who should get the HPV vaccine?

The CDC recommends HPV vaccination for women under age twenty-six and men under age twenty-one. They also recommended it for people who engage in anal sex, are transgender, or have weakened immune systems after age twenty-six, if they didn't get vaccinated when they were younger.

In 2018, the FDA approved expanded use of the HPV vaccine for people ages twenty-seven through forty-five, regardless of whether they've already had HPV, so be sure to ask your healthcare provider if you qualify.

adrienne maree brown

on realizing birth control wasn't designed for her body

In 2015, I had an ectopic pregnancy.

I was raised to believe sex was scary and dangerous, that any interaction could leave me with an STI or an unwanted pregnancy. Yet at some point in my mid-thirties, I realized, in spite of the fear, I needed that experience—I needed to feel what it was like to have sex with a man without anything between us. I'm pansexual, and I'll admit, I'm not as vigilant about contraception with people who can't get me pregnant.

I asked an eager old friend—someone I definitely didn't want to have a kid with—to have sex. We were both freshly tested. I intended to trust the rest of the protection to Plan B. After our fun, we went together to Duane Reade, purchased Plan B, then hugged goodbye. I took the pill, experienced some cramping the next day, and got what appeared to be a period after a week.

A month later, as I was opening a window in my home, I experienced the most intense pain I've ever felt, coming from the middle of my body. I knew I only had a few minutes to decide how I was going to survive—it was that kind of pain. Luckily, a friend arrived at that moment for tea and drove me to the hospital. They had me pee in a cup—excruciating. Shockingly, I was pregnant.

In the next few hours I endured one painful experience after another. I wasn't allowed to take any painkillers because there was a small chance the pregnancy could be saved. A nurse needed to perform an intravaginal ultrasound, and I am still very sorry for the things I said to her.

Once they had confirmed I had an ectopic pregnancy, that a misguided little life had attached itself to my left fallopian tube, and I had a significant amount of internal bleeding, they decided to operate. I was told I was very lucky that this happened at this moment in history. Fifty years ago, I wouldn't have survived. I was told this was a very, very rare situation, that the chances for someone like me—who rarely sleeps with men, who only slept with this one that one day, who took Plan B, to then have an ectopic pregnancy—were one in a million.

When I woke up after the surgery, I was told everything they had removed from my body had been disposed of as medical waste. I'm still sad about that, because I would have loved to have done a ritual for my loss. It took months for me to turn and face the grief.

During those foggy numb months, I was billed $25,000 for the procedure.

And I had the thoughts that I think many people have in the face of lost pregnancies: *What's wrong with me? What's wrong with my body? Am I not capable of carrying life?*

Many years later, I was watching a television show, *Shrill* (2019), where the main character experiences a pregnancy even after taking emergency contraception. She learns the Plan B pill is only at its most effective for bodies up to 175 pounds—much less than I weighed when I went into that Duane Reade.

I knew instantly that this piece of information would haunt me for the rest of my life. If I had been given a dose of Plan B that aligned with my weight, would I have gone through that horrific pain, would I have lost a fallopian tube?

I'll never know. I want to make sure all people understand that medicine is not always created with all bodies in mind. Especially Black bodies. I want us all to demand that our bodies are treated accurately, rather than wasting time and resources, and opening ourselves up to more tragedy.

I'm still learning. And I'm scared. But I hope my vulnerability will help others consider who benefits—and which systems benefit—when our needs and safety are not attended to.

adrienne is a writer, social justice facilitator, pleasure activist, healer, and doula living in Detroit. She is the author of *Emergent Strategy: Shaping Change, Changing Worlds* and *Pleasure Activism: The Politics of Feeling Good*, the coeditor of *Octavia's Brood: Science Fiction Stories from Social Justice Movements*, and cohost of the podcast *How to Survive the End of the World*. adrienne has been facilitating professionally for over 15 years, and has worked with hundreds of organizations, including informal collectives, foundations, and national networks.

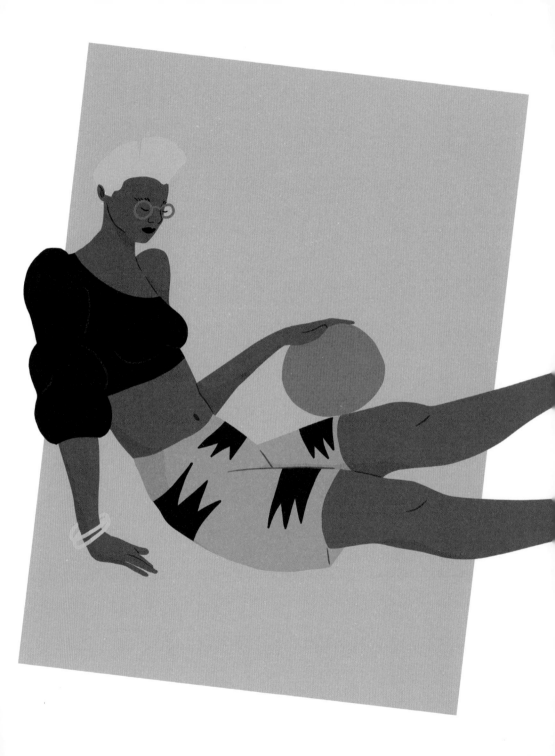

the sex ed you weren't taught

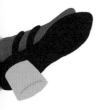

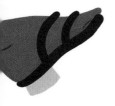

Perhaps you remember a health teacher showing you gross pictures of STIs. Or maybe you were in an abstinence-only program, where the instructor passed around a piece of tape until it lost its stickiness, likening it to a person who has multiple sex partners. (Because virgins are . . . sticky? The metaphor doesn't quite work.) Or, possibly, you had that class where you had to carry around a creepy robot baby for 48 hours to help you imagine how hard your life would be as a teen parent.

Sex ed curriculums vary wildly, but even the most progressive programs—the ones that affirm queer identities, foster open communication, and refrain from scare tactics—usually still fall short of tackling a few key topics. It's time to take a hard look at what we are (and are not) teaching young people about sex, and think about how we can set them up to have healthy sexual and romantic relationships.

consent

The #MeToo movement and other advocacy efforts have moved the topic of sexual consent into the national spotlight. But confusion remains in many circles about what consent actually looks like, how to communicate it, and when it's needed. So, let's clear those questions up, in the way they should have been in middle school.

Consent is an active, ongoing, enthusiastic expression of desire to engage in an activity. Consent is not the absence of "no," cold body language, saying "I'm not sure," or saying "yes" while drunk or under coercion. Legally speaking, a person is not able to give consent if they are under the influence of drugs or alcohol, or under the age of consent (which varies by state). Learning how to ask for, recognize, and give consent requires communication and emotional maturity. If you're too uncomfortable to talk to a partner about whether they're ready for sex and what type of sex they're interested in, you're probably not ready to have sex.

Developing a healthy understanding of consent also requires breaking down some traditional attitudes toward sex. The idea that sex is something men try to "get" and women have to protect against, for example, takes away agency from both parties, and ignores queer identities altogether. In reality, sex is not a reward that anyone can earn in exchange for being nice to another person or anything that one person owes to another. Healthy sex is wanted and enjoyed by all parties involved.

Asking for consent can be simple, but it requires truly listening to the other person's answer and monitoring your own behavior. For example, you can ask, "Can I kiss you right now?" and the person might say yes, but their tense body language says otherwise. That means you should stop what you're doing and check in with them. It's also important that if someone says "no" to an activity or touch, you respect their wishes. Asking for something again and again until the person gives in is a form of coercion. (Don't do that!)

Everyone also has the right to leave a situation that makes them uncomfortable in any way. You never have to have sex to prove you have strong feelings for someone, or because you've had sex with them before, or because you're in a relationship. If you don't want to have sex, you don't have to, and anyone who tries to tell you otherwise is not worthy of your time.

queer sex

The type of sex you're interested in might not be represented in your curriculum at all. Many sex ed programs prioritize safer practices and issues related to heterosexual sex, leaving queer kids on their own to figure out how to navigate their sexuality, what sex looks like for them, and how to stay safe.

Research shows that children are aware of their gender identity as young as age four—meaning that discussions of gender identity are an age-appropriate and necessary part of sexuality education. It can be life-affirming for gender-expansive kids to know that they aren't alone in their experiences and to have the language they need to describe their identities.

There are some key ideas that, if included in mainstream sex education, would go a long way toward ensuring every student gets the information they need.

There are three parts of a person's gender: body, identity, and expression. All these parts operate independently.

1. *Body* refers to your anatomy—how your body functions, how bodies are gendered by society, and how others interact with you based on your body.

2. *Identity* comes from your internal, deeply understood sense of self. For some people, gender identity matches up with their body; this is known as being *cisgender*. For others, it doesn't match, which is sometimes known as being *transgender*, or, more broadly, *gender expansive*.

3. *Expression* is how you style and present yourself to the world.

Gender exists on a spectrum, with identities like genderfluid and nonbinary existing in addition to male and female.

Gender is also completely separate from sexual orientation—gender has to do with who you are, while sexual orientation describes who you are attracted to romantically and sexually. Sex refers to any activity in which someone is trying to achieve an orgasm. Penis-in-vagina sex is not the only thing that qualifies as sex, nor is it the only sex act with associated risks. Most humans are also somewhere on a spectrum of sexual orientation, not exclusively gay or straight. One person in a hundred is asexual, meaning they have no sexual attraction to anyone.

the role of pleasure

Learning the role of sex in procreation and how to have safer sex is critical, but these conversations often dance around the whole point of why humans have sex most of the time: because it feels good.

Middle and high school classrooms can feel like the last place anyone might want to discuss sexual pleasure (like, *awkward*), but these lessons are key in setting up young people to have mutually fulfilling sexual relationships. In some spaces, the idea that sex is supposed to feel good *for all parties involved* can be revolutionary.

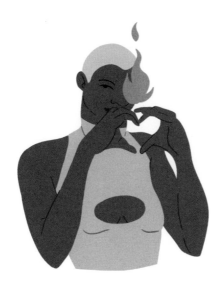

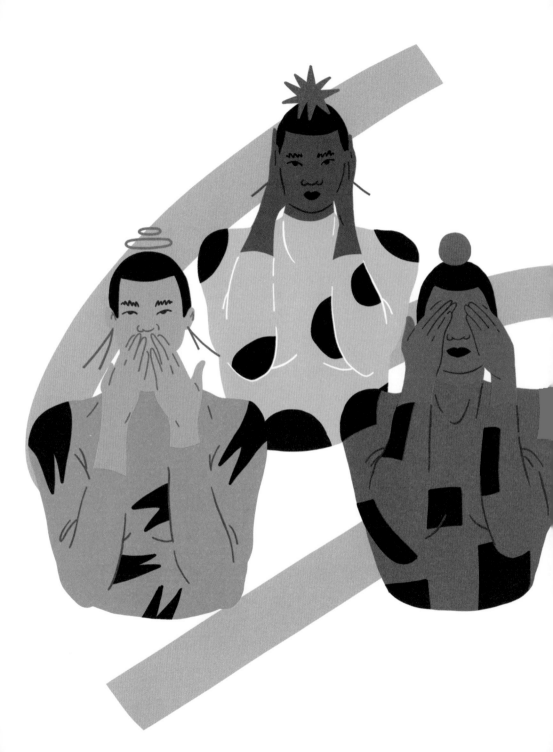

the weirdest things we used to believe about sex

Puberty is a wild time, filled with moments of learning, realization, and . . . crushing amounts of shame. The shame can be at least 50 percent attributed to the fact that, in our pubescent years, we're all trying to find the answers to the greatest mystery of them all (sex) without actually having to talk to anybody about it. And no thanks to sex ed, of course! Seriously, if you haven't already, give yourself a pat on the back for eventually figuring all (or most) of it out. Check out what a few of our younger selves used to believe about doin' the do.

Thanks to *Where Did I Come From?* by Dr. Spock, I knew pretty early on that sex was for making babies, and it happened when a penis entered a vagina and sperm met with an egg. But did the penis go into the vagina and just kinda hang out there? What was the incentive to even do such an odd-seeming thing? In middle school, I flipped to a page in my best friend's mom's handbook on being a woman and found sex positions for pregnant people—and the whole sex-for-pleasure realization exploded into my world.

—Laura B.

The weirdest thing I used to believe about sex was that it didn't count unless it involved a penis entering a vagina. Ha, how much I've learned.

—Sam P.

I never really had "the talk" with anyone, so like any hormonal teenager with a Wi-Fi connection, I turned to the internet for answers. My period was late, and I'd recently done the scandalous deed of holding hands with a boy, so naturally, I googled the two things together. One internet black hole later, and after some anonymous commenter on a message board had convinced me that semen could come out of fingertips, I knew I was absolutely, positively, 100 percent pregnant. Fingertips, friends. A few lessons I learned here: Periods can be irregular from time to time, correlation is not necessarily causation, and no matter what the internet says, it is biologically impossible for anyone to impregnate you with their hands.

—Rachel C.

I used to think that using lube was basically the equivalent of admitting defeat, and that there must be something wrong with me if we ever needed that.

—Morgan R.

I used to believe women could get pregnant by sitting on a dirty toilet because I heard it on *The Ricki Lake Show* in 1998. Thanks, Ricki.

—Kathleen A.

So, I took the phrase "popping the cherry" super literally. Like I thought it was a real thing, like how Anne Hathaway pops her foot in *The Princess Diaries*. But when you actually have sex for the first time, literally nothing happens, and nothing pops at all. I was almost disappointed.

—Carolyn K.

Before I hit puberty, I used to think that when I masturbated (and orgasmed), it was going to encourage my period to come (no pun intended) faster. And obviously, I didn't want that because I didn't want to get caught! I missed out on years of orgasms because I was too afraid of starting my period before the right time and my mom finding out why.

—Dani B.

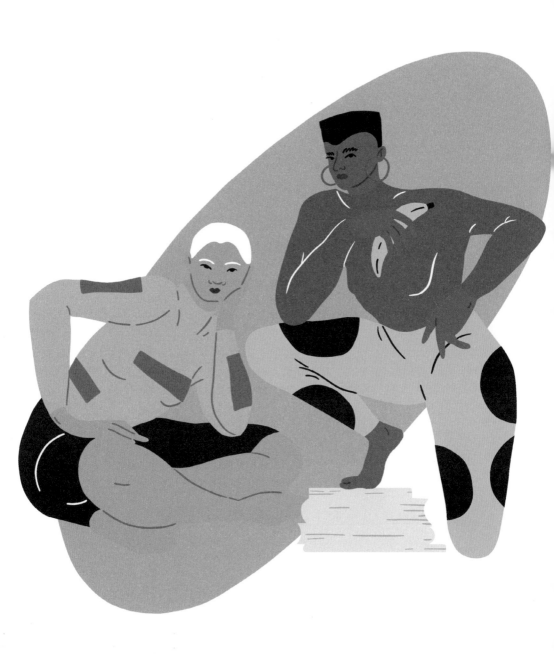

the state of sex ed policy

For many of us in the United States, the phrase "sex ed" conjures a picture of our middle school gym teacher, fast-talking through a vague description of heterosexual sex before fumbling a brandless condom onto a banana. We see this image in teen movies, punchlines, and pop culture at large.

But sexual education in the US can take dozens of different forms, since there is no federal regulation of such programs. This means states can choose whether to require sex ed and what topics to cover. Some schools offer broad sexuality education programs that start teaching about consent and communication in kindergarten. Others promote abstinence-only sex ed, passing around visual aids like chewing gum or a spit-filled cup to demonstrate how someone who has multiple partners can become "contaminated." The research about what works is clear: Comprehensive, judgment-free sex ed results in lower rates of teen pregnancy and STI transmission. Furthermore, students who have participated in comprehensive sex ed have their first sexual encounter at a later age than those who have received abstinence-only sex ed, or none at all.

And yet, stalwart resistance to comprehensive, inclusive sex ed programs continues in many areas of the country. Opponents are concerned that learning about sex will sexualize children too early, encourage promiscuous behavior, and even "promote homosexuality."

These debates around sex ed cut deep; for most folks with strong feelings about these programs (either for or against), their perspectives are inextricably linked to their identity, morality, and religious beliefs. It's a tricky topic many politicians don't want to touch—which is why the US is left with inadequate and outdated laws about sexual education.

state by state

Sex ed requirements in the US range from no requirements on the books (as in Idaho), to mandated, medically accurate, culturally relevant gender and sexuality-inclusive programs (California). In the US overall, 24 states and Washington, DC, mandate sex education; 13 require the instruction to be medically accurate; 8 require it to be unbiased against any race, gender, or ethnicity; and 2 prohibit it from promoting religion.

the impact

These varied requirements mean that young people may not receive any formal sexual education in school, or will receive information that is incomplete or biased. Whether or not the sex ed a student receives is relevant to their sexual orientation, cultural context, or social reality depends on where they live. These issues disproportionately affect students in less affluent districts, whose optional sex ed programs are more likely to get cut by funding issues, as well as students of color and LGBTQ+ students, who are less likely to see their experiences represented in curricula that prioritize white, heterosexual, cisgender experiences.

As of 2019, 6 states have homophobia written into their sex ed laws. Alabama, Louisiana, Mississippi, Oklahoma, South Carolina, and Texas all have laws that prohibit the mention of homosexual relationships, apart from teaching that gay sex is associated with AIDS. The Alabama law even includes the false statement that homosexuality is illegal. The existence of trans and nonbinary gender identities is not mentioned in any of these requirements, which translates to those topics being left out of the discussion at many schools. This lack of representation, or outright shaming of queer experiences, can have profoundly negative effects. LGBTQ+ students have higher instances of anxiety, depression, and bullying when they go to a school that does not include queer topics in its curricula.

Students of color are often excluded from sex ed as well. Abstinence-only programs, known to be less effective, are concentrated in schools with the highest numbers of students of color. And even in schools that do provide comprehensive programs, the information might not be as relevant to the lived experiences of students of color. Sexual expectations, pressures, and attitudes vary depending on a young person's racial and cultural background. Young girls of color, for example, tend to be seen as more mature, more sexual, and less innocent than white girls their age. And a recent study found that young Black men are more likely than other racial groups to have sex before age thirteen—due in part to a failure of sex ed programs to address the social pressure and expectations that are specific to young Black men. Health research also has an ugly history of racism, particularly as it relates to eugenics and fertility, but that information is often left out of curricula.

The fact that most sex ed programs ignore the ways that culture and identity interact with bodies and sex means that a large portion of our young people are not receiving the information they need to make empowered choices.

around the world

On the most basic level, young people around the world need access to comprehensive sex education so they can make informed decisions about their health and well-being. But, even on a global scale, sex ed policy still has a long way to go.

According to the Guttmacher Institute, in countries like Peru, Kenya, and Ghana, there is no policy that mandates comprehensive sex education. A study in

2017 found that in Peru alone, 3 in 4 teachers lack the materials they need to teach sexual education—which translates to a majority of students missing out on much-needed information about their changing bodies.

How much or how little sexual health and education are prioritized can depend on the cultural or religious values of a country, and on the fact that the US often sets the pace for global advancements (or lack thereof). If the US is dragging its feet on policy changes, chances are that many other countries are at even more of a standstill. (Meanwhile, the Netherlands is ahead of the game, with truly comprehensive sex education beginning when students are four years old.) The good news is that many organizations are committed to making sure *all* people are empowered with sexual health and wellness information. The World Association for Sexual Health and the International Planned Parenthood Federation are devoted to promoting sexual education and intervention tactics for marginalized populations, like members of the queer community, displaced people and refugees, and racial and ethnic minorities. Change takes time, but no matter the obstacles, there are many people and institutions committed to seeing it through.

the fight for inclusivity

In the US, advocates in many states are fighting to make sexual education policies more inclusive, either by appealing to lawmakers for new legislation or creating their own programs entirely. Organizations like Advocates for Youth and Planned Parenthood offer a variety of programs and resources for educators, parents, and young people to learn how to start healthy conversations about sex. Several state legislatures are currently locked in debates about whether to pass more inclusive sex ed bills, ones that push for open, honest conversations about bodies and relationships. And organizations like Philly-based Daughters of the Diaspora are fighting for sex ed that better serves young people of color. If you're fired up about making sex ed more comprehensive, inclusive, and accessible, supporting any of these groups is a good way to jump into the fight.

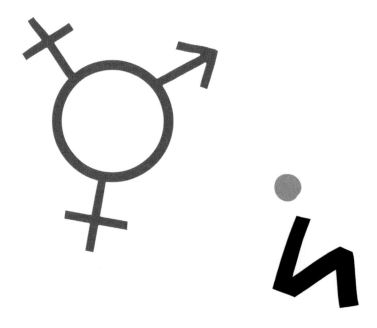

Liara Roux

on why social justice can't leave
sex workers behind

For a long time, I kept my politics at arm's length from my work. As a sex worker, I figured I would make more money if I kept things fun and sexy—I didn't want to scare off potential clients with my political screeds! But in October 2017, after Patreon (a crowdfunding membership platform) and other tech companies started to crack down on sex workers and adjacent sexual content on their platforms, I became scared for my future. More than that, I was scared for my friends. As a white sex worker who advertises online and is usually read as a cis woman,

I was able to figure out alternative payment options. This wasn't the case for one of my friends, a trans woman living in Central America. She had just started making enough to sign a lease on a new apartment; if Patreon kicked her off, she didn't know how she would survive.

It seemed sex workers were being forced off the internet; I had my Twitter account suspended, and around a thousand sex workers reported their accounts were banned from Instagram. Together with a group of organizers, I made a massive list detailing all the companies that would not allow sex workers on their platforms. That list was longer than I could have imagined. Being apolitical was no longer an option. I had to engage to survive.

Sex and pleasure are powerful motivators; part of why the patriarchy is powerful and self-sustaining is because it controls access to sex and pleasure. Who is allowed to feel pleasure during sex? Under what circumstances is sex legally and morally acceptable? Historically, sexual norms were often dictated by religious leaders. Those who strayed outside their decrees were considered immoral. Even kings had to be concerned— King Henry VIII famously wrested control of the Church of England from papal authority so he could divorce his wife and marry another woman he found desirable.

Sex workers are mediators of pleasure. In the United States, the dominant social norm is that the wife should be the sole source of sexual pleasure for her husband. A man directing his resources to a person who is not his wife in exchange for pleasure is inherently destabilizing to the traditional nuclear family. Unlike the traditional housewife, most sex workers are not reliant on any one partner for their financial security. Sex workers are often women, queer folk, and other marginalized identities. Giving these communities independent sources of income terrifies those who benefit from heteronormative, white supremacist, patriarchal power structures. Why? It has the potential to destroy them.

As a result, they are trying to destroy sex workers' rights first. We are denied housing, medical treatment, banking services . . . the list goes on. If we are to survive, we need allies to fight stigma and discrimination. The next time you hear someone make a joke about "dead hookers," explain to them why that's dehumanizing. Give money to direct aid organizations, like St. James Infirmary, which provides medical care to the sex work community. Advocate for dismantling the carceral justice system. Read books and blog posts and Twitter threads written by sex workers about sex workers. Ask the candidates you vote for if they support sex workers' rights, and if they don't, explain to them why decriminalization is important.

Most importantly: Pay your sex workers! No more pirated porn. If you're invested in fighting inequality, stepping up for sex workers' rights is imperative.

Liara is a sex worker, an independent adult media producer and director, and a political organizer focused on freedom of sexual expression, as well as the decriminalization and protection of consensual adult activity.

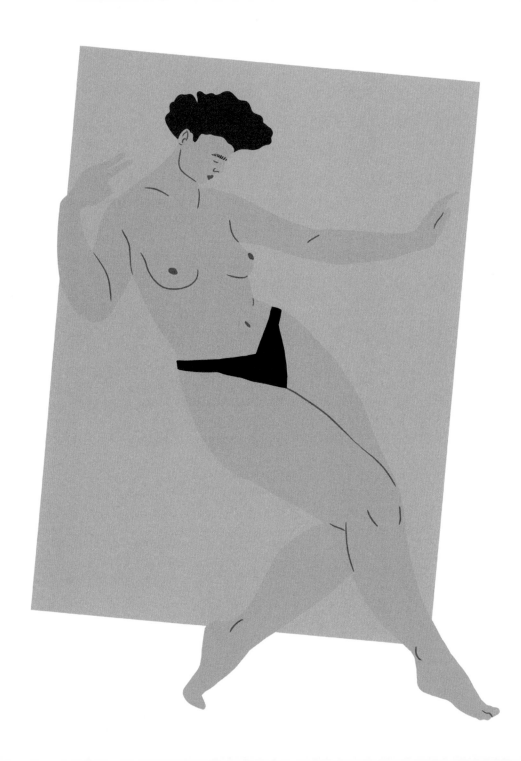

stopping revenge porn

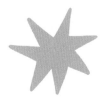

Sharing intimate photos within consensual relationships is a pretty popular and normal occurrence, given the amount of time and effort we put into interacting with people who aren't present. We've seen the words "revenge porn" (also called nonconsensual pornography, or NCP) on television and in media outlets for a significant amount of time now, and the frequency is partly due to our ability to access content and share information with one simple click. In the legal world, revenge porn constitutes nonconsensual pornography and is defined as the distribution of sexually graphic images of individuals without their consent. This includes taking compromising images or videos of someone without their knowledge, as well as sharing material recorded within an intimate, consensual relationship. Like other emotionally damaging invasions of privacy and personal attacks, such as sexual assault and intimate partner violence, nonconsensual porn brings trauma, victim-blaming, and shame.

It also highlights a legal system that has yet to reflect the times and adopt laws that can protect one's privacy in the abyss that is the World Wide Web. Often, leaked nude photos garner more public shame for women than men—we've seen this imbalance with some of our favorite stars, including Rihanna, Jennifer Lawrence, and Miley Cyrus. In these scenarios, when photos of female celebrities were leaked, the victims suffered humiliation and tarnished images, whereas when male celebrity nude photos were leaked (there aren't very many—to be honest), it's a source of humor or even praise, and it rarely negatively affects the trajectory of their careers.

Then, there's the obvious question, "Why send nude selfies if you don't want people to see them?" These kinds of questions wrongly shift the burden and blame onto the victim. It is never the victim's fault. The shame women can feel in these situations is *so* real. Even if you know you did nothing wrong, the fact that there are photos of you at your most vulnerable, on the internet, distributed without your consent, can make you feel powerless and ashamed. Revenge porn is used as a potent weapon and can follow victims for a long time. These photos and images can be exposed to future romantic partners or employers from a simple internet search.

how is this being legislated?

Prosecuting nonconsensual porn varies wildly from country to country. German law, for example, gives people the right to "revoke consent" at any time, which requires any party to whom they distributed personal photos to delete them. Whereas in the US, only some states have nonconsensual porn laws that make sharing these images a crime. The reality of the crime and its prosecution is a whole lot more complicated. Only in February of 2019 did New York State pass a bill to outlaw revenge porn, joining forty-six other states (plus DC and Guam) that passed similar legislation. It hasn't been an easy feat—judges have often turned down court appeals on the grounds of free speech. Under most of these laws, the offender can serve up to 1 year in jail (or 3 years of probation) and is required to remove all of the illegal content from their social media platforms. Minors can also be prosecuted in family court, and in more serious cases, the offender will have to register on the sex offenders list. Jail might sound extreme, but in countries like Denmark, Israel, Japan, and the Philippines, offenders can be incarcerated for up to 5 years for distributing revenge porn.

These efforts to control how private images are shared online stem from the larger question of the role government plays in regulating social media. Many larger technology companies initially pushed back on this legislation in order to not be held liable for content that is published on their platforms. The happy medium was to only hold the culprit financially responsible—not these companies—but still require the companies to remove any content that was published without consent (when asked).

what can people do to protect their private images?

There are some precautions we can all take to avoid giving someone else the power to share our private images. Most of our cell phones are connected to the internet in some way or another. In order to guarantee mobile pictures don't make it online, try to avoid taking compromising photos. If you do, keep them for your own personal collection and refrain from sending them to others. While some friendships and relationships may appear to be forever, you just never know! They don't call it "revenge" porn for nothing. Try to keep your face out of pictures, or use apps with temporary pictures that expire after a certain amount of time—although even that isn't foolproof! It's also important to be firm and serious with others about taking photos and videos you do not approve of.

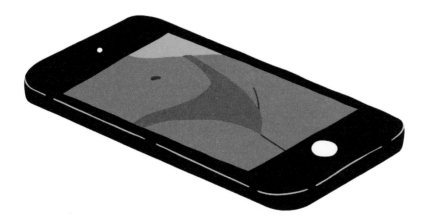

what should you do if your images surface online?

First off, don't panic.

Take screenshots of all images and any offensive communication between yourself and the culprit. Do a reverse image search to try to find as many versions and copies of the images as possible. You will need this as evidence if you decide to take legal action.

Respond as quickly as possible by alerting authorities (if it's illegal in your state to publish NCP) or seeking guidance. The Cyber Civil Rights Initiative is a platform that offers a 24-hour crisis hotline as well as emotional and technical support to cyber victims.

Report the NCP to the various social media platforms. Google, Facebook, Twitter, Instagram, Reddit, and Tumblr will remove NCP images once reported. Make sure you take the time to report the image across all sites.

Your sexual privacy, whether online or in the comfort of your own bedroom, should never be compromised!

why access to abortion must be protected

Dr. Jenn Conti

No matter how much anyone proselytizes, abortion is not a straightforward issue. I know this because I am an abortion provider, but way before that, I considered myself to be "pro-life." I've looked at abortion from all angles and have spent innumerable hours dissecting every element of why it has been such a divisive ideological issue throughout time and geography. History has largely shaped the modern abortion discussion, and it's important to realize this idea of abortion as a gray area used to be a lot more popular. In 1973, when the landmark US Supreme Court case *Roe v. Wade* legalized abortion nationwide, Justice Harry Blackmun acknowledged this in the Court's majority opinion.

He wrote:

"We need not resolve the difficult question of when life begins. When those trained in the respective disciplines of medicine, philosophy, and theology are unable to arrive at any consensus, the judiciary, at this point in the development of man's knowledge, is not in a position to speculate as to the answer."

Even as they decided the legality of abortion in America, the Court wasn't going to touch the morality issue with a ten-foot pole. This is because even a bipartisan court of all white men knew that regardless of personal, religious, moral, or philosophical beliefs, public health mattered most.

Access to abortion is a life-saving service that studies have shown irrefutably decreases maternal mortality. In countries like Romania, South Africa, and Nepal, maternal mortality rates plummeted following national liberalizations of abortion laws, and all without increasing the incidence of abortion. The opposite is true of countries who have tightened their abortion restrictions: The number of pregnant women dying soars. So why, then, are we still fighting this fight? Why is abortion access even an issue?

Here's the answer: misogyny (and racism, as a bonus). There is an ugly, deep-rooted, and ingrained prejudice against women (if not outright oppression) throughout all parts of the world; with that comes inflexible perspectives, or the refusal to conceptualize the complexity of living with an undesired pregnancy. As a result, abortion access is rapidly eroding in the US.

In the first half of 2019, fifteen US states (FL, GA, IL, KY, LA, MD, MN, MS, MO, NY, OH, SC, TN, TX, WV) introduced bills to criminalize abortion as early as 6 weeks into a pregnancy, or only 2 weeks after a missed period (assuming you have an average, 28-day menstrual cycle). Most people don't even realize they're pregnant that early, especially if they have irregular cycles, which upwards of 35 percent of women do, according to recent data. These "heartbeat bills," as anti-choice proponents have misleadingly branded them, are some of the most rigid laws posed, aiming to essentially wipe out abortion altogether, given their cutoff points. And while anti-abortion restrictions are certainly not new, the gusto and emboldened nature of more recent laws is something to be feared. When conservative Brett Kavanaugh replaced Justice Anthony Kennedy in 2018, the Supreme Court was stacked to finally challenge the constitutionality of *Roe v. Wade.* The harmful restrictions that preceded Kavanaugh's appointment—target regulation of abortion provider (TRAP) laws, 48- and 72-hour waiting limits, parental consent laws, bans on medication abortion, and more— were child's play compared to "heartbeat bills."

Bill HB481 in Georgia goes further than simply banning abortion after the time at which a fetal heartbeat can be detected. It threatens to imprison people who terminate their pregnancies, as well as the doctors who perform abortions. It grants full legal personhood to fetuses, ensuring a person who gets or gives an abortion would be prosecuted for murder; prosecutes people who leave the state to terminate their pregnancy elsewhere; and allows prosecutors to investigate those who miscarry.

The legal crafting of these laws is vile but also strategic and well planned. It is not an accident that cutthroat laws like this are spewing out of Southern states, where people (and especially people of color) are already familiar with limited abortion access. To be clear, abortion may be legal in the United States, but that doesn't mean it's accessible. There is only one abortion clinic in the entire state of Mississippi, and TRAP laws threaten to similarly reduce access in Louisiana, as well as other states. When HB2 passed in Texas in 2013, access essentially disappeared for thousands of women as TRAP laws halved the number of abortion clinics from over forty to only nineteen.

The small victories that once ensured abortion access, like the 2016 SCOTUS ruling on *Whole Woman's Health v. Hellerstedt* (which overturned HB2), are no longer protective or reassuring. It's an entirely different landscape when legal precedent doesn't matter, when politicians play doctor, and when we do not value people with vaginas as equal beings. Regardless, we will keep on fighting.

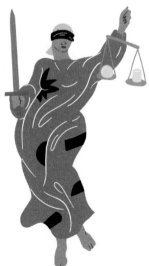

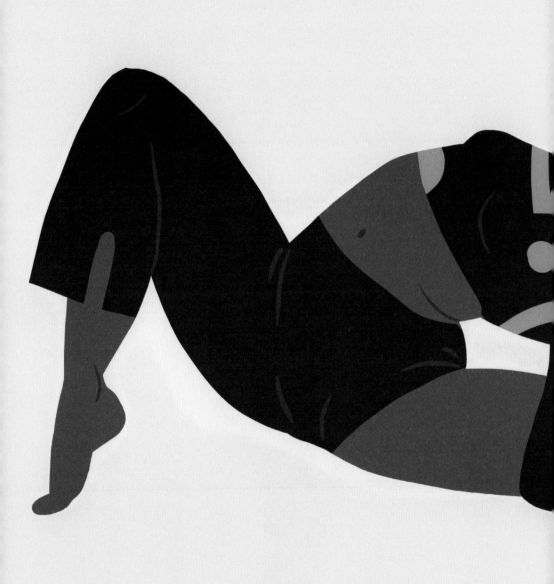

CHAPTER 4

wellness & self-care

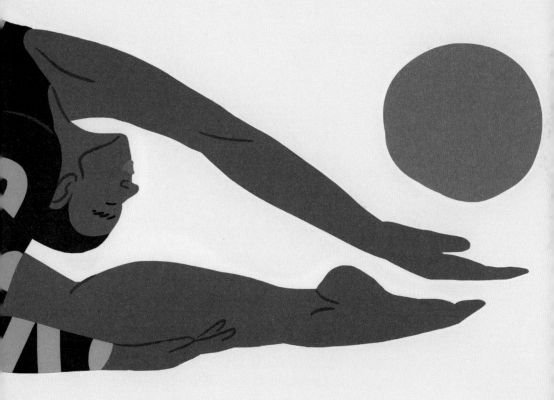

the benefits of exercising on your period

For a long time, people with periods were told to avoid a whole bunch of things while they were menstruating, and the reasons why were—surprise—pretty much made up. One of those things? Physical activity of any kind.

While we now know that we're allowed to do whatever we damn well want, it's understandable why you might be inclined to skip your weekly spin class during your period. (Seriously, doing "whatever we damn well want" definitely still includes opting out of physical activity of any kind, don't worry.) However, there are a few pros to hitting the gym during your period week that might be worth considering. And if you're feeling bloaty and bleh, remember that every workout doesn't have to be intense! Opt for slower, low-impact exercises like yoga, Pilates, or walking to the store that's kinda far from your apartment but carries the ice cream you like (it counts, OK?).

Just be mindful that you're not over-exerting your body—take the breaks you need, and don't ever try to push through pain. Here are some of the benefits of keeping things active while you flow.

fight fatigue

Chances are, your period has left you feeling a little sluggish. While you probably want to go about your day as slowly as possible, subverting your body's instincts can give you the boost you need.

The reason you're usually exhausted during your period in the first place is because your hormones go all over the place once your body realizes it doesn't have to continue developing an environment for a potential fetus. And as we all know, your hormone levels have the power to mess with a whole bunch of things going on in your body, and these changes (all happening rapidly) are tiring AF.

Regular exercise, on the other hand, can naturally balance your hormone levels. Also, keep in mind that your body will yield the best, most consistent results when workouts are a part of your normal routine.

ease your cramps

When you're getting into the groove of a good workout, your body releases tiny neurotransmitters called endorphins. They're a natural painkiller and they're the best. Endorphins are so effective, a couple studies even show that they could be an effective pain reliever for people giving birth, which is pretty metal. Getting your heart rate up also increases blood circulation, doing wonders for period-week aches in your abdomen and lower back.

naturally boost your mood

As Harvard scholar Elle Woods once said, "Endorphins make you happy. Happy people just don't shoot their husbands!" Let's focus on that first part: The same hormones that will keep you from reaching for another cup of coffee at 2 p.m. also deliver a nice li'l boost to your mood.

The best part is, if high-intensity workouts aren't your thing, you can still reap the benefits of low-intensity workouts; doing a long workout will also do the trick. The mood boost from these endorphins is referred to as a "runner's high."

maximize your workouts

You might be surprised to hear your period week could be the most efficient time for you to hit the gym. According to a study from Umeå University in Sweden, women who worked out on their period reported increased muscle mass and greater overall strength than when they worked out during other weeks of their cycle.

Despite these benefits, don't forget to check in with yourself. If you have pain that gets worse or you start to feel nauseous or dizzy at any point during your workout, Stop! Hydrate! Know your body and its limits.

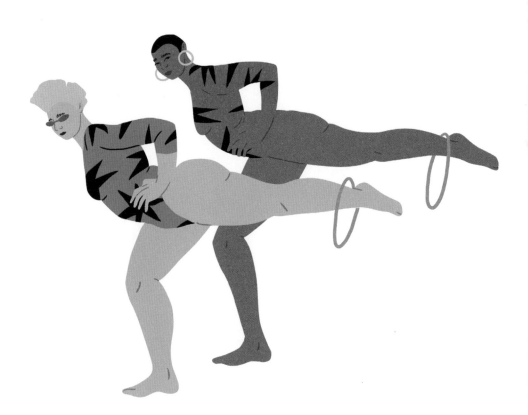

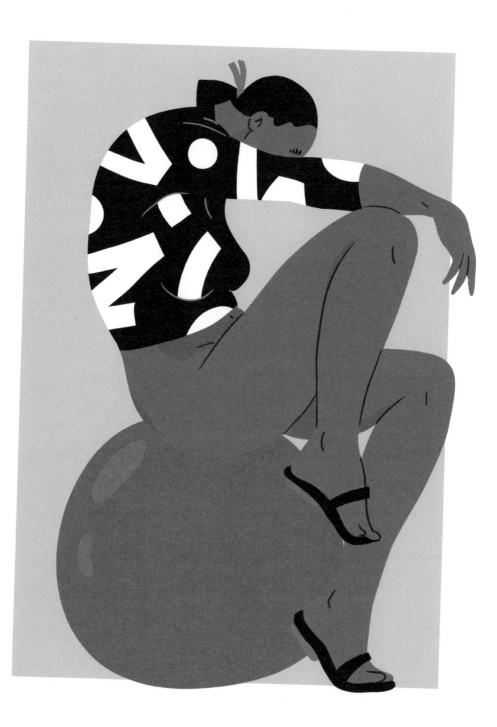

caring for your hair down there

Just like the hair on your head, all the hair on your body should get a little TLC, especially if it's on an important, sensitive area like your vulva. Yup, let's talk about pubes.

Whether you have a strict running appointment with a waxer who you also consider your best friend or you go au naturel, there is absolutely no wrong way to wear your hair down there. (And hey, maybe anyone who thinks they deserve an opinion on your pubes doesn't deserve access to your vagina. Just a thought!) What does matter is that your grooming methods are safe, protect you from unwanted infections, and ideally are not motivated by patriarchal ideals.

is pubic hair dirty?

No, it's not. The misconception that body hair is unhygienic in general is as old as time, even though it's really just an aesthetic choice. Seriously, dating back to 2 BC, the Roman poet Ovid encouraged women to remove their body hair so "that no rude goat find his way beneath your arms, and that your legs be not rough with bristling hairs." Interestingly enough, there are far fewer quotes that have stood the test of time that express this concern for male bodies. Go figure!

Wait (you might be thinking), so is it actually unhealthy to go bare? Don't worry, as long as you're practicing proper hygiene, your vagina will be happy and healthy. However, there are a few things you should keep in mind to make sure you're trimming (or plucking or waxing or lasering) your hedges safely.

preventing and removing ingrown hairs

Curly or coarse hair that's been shaved is especially prone to becoming ingrown. If you notice you're getting a lot of ingrown hairs down there, you might want to try switching hair removal methods. You could also try exfoliating regularly and making sure you're practicing safe shaving (more on that in a sec).

Already got an ingrown? Stop. Put down the tweezers and back away slowly. The temptation to go to town on an ingrown hair is not worth a potentially very nasty infection. If the hair is partially above your skin, you can carefully pluck it with clean tweezers, but if not—resist! Avoid doing any more hair removal in that area until the ingrown goes away (which it should do on its own). If you're antsy, applying warm compresses to the area a few times a day can speed up the process. If the hair is being particularly stubborn, consult your doctor, who can recommend a topical cream to clear things up.

wax like a pro

If you do opt for waxing, you should just go to a pro, first making sure the facility is legit. (This is decidedly not the time for bargain hunting!) Checking out internet reviews or asking your friends for recommendations is a good place to start, but you should go to any prospective salon in person and check it out. Look for cleanliness, of course, but it's a red flag if the waxers double-dip the wax applicators, unless they use a new pot of wax for every client and throw it out afterward. Reusing applicators can fast-track bacterial infections of all kinds.

After a wax, it's usually a good idea to avoid super-hot showers or baths, scented soaps or lotions, and sex. Your vulva is a trooper; let the area chill out and decompress for a second while any swelling goes down!

shaving safely

Shaving is one of the most popular methods of hair removal for a reason: It's cheap and doesn't require a trip to the salon. However, with great power comes great responsibility—below we've listed five tips for getting the job done without turning your bathroom into the opening scene of *Carrie*.

1. Buy razors marketed to men. They're straight up just better at removing hair (and also cheaper for some reason). It's very unfair, we know.

2. Never dry shave, and always prep first. Rinse the area with warm water to open up your pores, then trim long hair first. Apply shaving cream or hair conditioner (if you really truly actually must in a pinch). Either is better than soap for your skin.

3. Hold your skin taut and shave toward the direction your hair grows, not against. If you're prone to ingrowns, this tip should be non-negotiable. You shouldn't pass over the same spot more than once.

4. Take your time. (Ideally, you shouldn't be rushing to shave 20 minutes before a date.)

5. After you're done, rinse the area with cold water to close the pores back up. This will help prevent clogged and irritated skin.

ASK DR. JENN

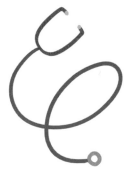

does my gyno care how much hair is down there?

The short answer is no. You do you when it comes to your pubic hair. Here's where we do care though: Shaving and waxing increase your chances of getting a skin infection in that area, which can be pretty gnarly. You don't want to be the person hospitalized for a pube-related infection from your vajazzling adventures. As long as you're staying safe, we don't care what you do with your hair.

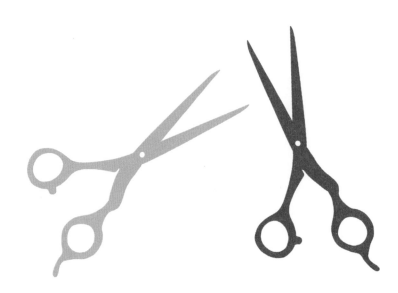

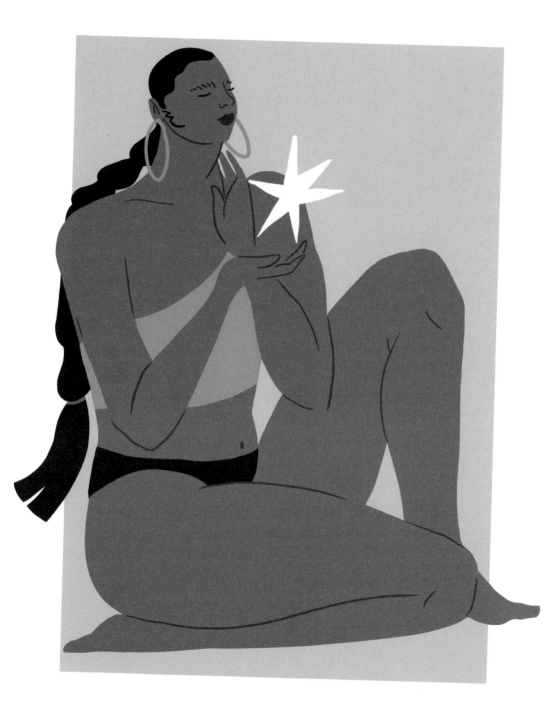

how hormones affect your skin

It's no secret that hormone fluctuations can create unwanted blemishes and skin irregularities, and throw off the texture and balance of your otherwise gorgeous skin, no matter how many sheet masks you do. We don't usually condone blaming your problems on your period, but in this case, have at it! It's common for your skin to break out anywhere from 7 to 10 days before your period, and you will likely be extra sensitive if you touch, pluck, or pop anything on your body. You can blame this tenderness on prostaglandins (a group of chemicals released as the uterine lining sheds), which cause inflammation in the skin and body as well as menstrual cramps. As with many things that exist in our bodies, it's all about balance. Generally, your estrogen levels are low on days 1 to 7 of your cycle, and highest around days 7 to 14. During menstruation, both hormones drop to their lowest levels, and then testosterone becomes the dominant hormone. Testosterone triggers your sebaceous glands to produce more oil, which in turn causes acne.

All hormonal birth control methods that have estrogen (like the pill, patch, and ring) decrease acne by increasing production of SHBG (sex hormone binding globulin) in your liver, which then acts to bind and inactivate any circulating testosterone. If your hormonal acne is somewhat manageable, you may be able to get by with topical retinoid gels, creams, and lotions. Having a chat with your gynecologist along with a dermatologist might be a good idea if you feel like you might need to call in the big guns.

follow a skin-care routine

Consistency is key when it comes to your skin-care routine, especially during PMS and the days leading up to your period. Try using a face wash with salicylic acid during that crucial time—especially if you're acne prone. Hormones might make your skin prone to oiliness and acne, but don't give it any help by leaving dirt on your face at the end of the day!

Where we place our faces during resting hours is just as important as how we treat our skin during the day. Maybe even more important, because sleeping is a crucial time for skin rejuvenation. Try to keep your hair contained, and change your pillowcases often—you don't want all of the oil, hair, dead skin, and more that's stuck in your pillow getting on your face while you're dreaming about crushing your goals.

what not to do

Steer clear of scrubs, other harsh acids, and intense cosmetic procedures. These treatments will only exacerbate your blemishes and make your skin more irritated. Instead, indulge in being extra gentle with your skin and body during your period. It's also best to stay away from using oils to cleanse the skin, as oils can clog your pores. It might be a good idea to try an oil-free moisturizer too.

Sun exposure is one of the most common offenders leading to not-so-perfect skin. Too much sun can increase wrinkles—which are not the worst thing in the world despite what every commercial you've ever seen says. But more importantly, too much sun puts you at risk for skin cancer. Skin cancer is the leading cancer in the US, and while it's pretty impossible to avoid the sun altogether, you can take the necessary precautions by lathering on at least SPF 30 sunscreen and reapplying frequently. Applying sunscreen should be a regular step in your skin-care routine, even beneath makeup.

Ingrid Nilsen

on why managing her mental health is a work in progress (and that's OK!)

My period never bothered me much when I was younger. Throughout my teens and most of my twenties, it was sometimes heavy and annoying but rarely painful. At thirty, everything changed. My periods became unpredictable and ruthless. My cramps are so piercing they keep me up at night—moving from my lower abdomen all the way up into my ribs. However, one of the most difficult things to manage is the mental and emotional toll.

The 2 weeks before my period feel like I'm being swallowed whole and thrown into a dark underbelly of existence. This place is a shell of my life that's cold and unforgiving. Before my last period, I picked a fight with my girlfriend for no reason—my monster of an imagination concocted something and served it up. Negative thoughts instantly become singular truths. The walls close in on me. I cry, and I cry, and I cry. The space gets smaller. I feel suffocated. I don't recognize myself at all.

How do you climb out of a hole when it feels like there's nothing to hold on to? I desperately wish face masks and spa treatments could be my cure, but they don't even come close. I've had to sink into a deeper level of self-care—the kind that requires complete surrender. First, I had to acknowledge what I feel is real and not made up. Our culture enjoys labeling people who menstruate as "crazy." A heightened emotional state often instigates the clichéd question: "Are you on your period?" Which is really just a passive-aggressive insult for stepping out of your pretty little good girl box.

The hardest part has been being honest with other people about how I'm feeling and taking responsibility for my actions. I'm afraid of going to the doctor because in the past, I've been judged harshly and not taken seriously. I will go eventually, but I have to work through that history and fear first. Going to therapy regularly has been a complete savior. I relish walking to my appointments, even when it's pouring rain, because it forces me to be present. Following my intuition has also been key—I'm amazed at how it's still there, even in the midst of trekking through emotional quicksand. Whether it tells me to move my body, slow down, or get an ice-cream cone, it's never wrong and it never fails me. The moment may be fleeting, but even the smallest amount of relief or delight is enough to keep me moving forward.

While I'm not in control of my hormonal fluctuations, I am in control of how I treat other people. That fight I picked with my girlfriend? I had to apologize and admit my behavior was not OK. I've had to ask for help, too. Sometimes when an especially dark cloud looms overhead, I just need to vent. Talking to friends who believe me and who share similar experiences has been incredibly healing—they ground me. And then, just when I feel like I'm making progress, my period comes. The darkness bleeds away. I'm me again—at least until next month.

Ingrid is an NYC-based creative and online video personality. With over 8 million followers across her social channels, Ingrid creates informative content using beauty and fashion as a starting point for deeper conversations. When she's not online, she's hanging out in Brooklyn with her dog and eating bagels.

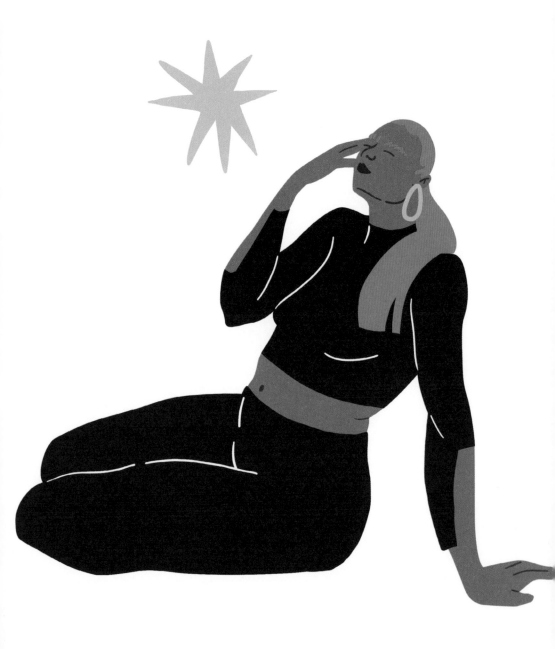

personalized acts of self-care

Between long work days and packed calendars, it can be surprisingly easy to forget about taking care of yourself. It might seem frivolous, but neglecting to slow down and simply rest every once in a while can lead to serious stress and burnout. We all know this, especially since #selfcare has been trending for years now (and for good reason), but we should definitely avoid just going through the motions. Self-care does and should mean different things to different people, and what works for one person may not work for another. Finding what personally relaxes you and helps you de-stress is important—but that doesn't mean you can't look to others for inspiration! Check out what a few friends had to say about their own personal acts of self-care.

Working in social media, this one doesn't fly all the time; however, whenever I know someone else can cover me on emails or when it's a slow day, I just turn off my phone for my commute home. Not just put it on airplane mode, but 100 percent shut it down. I have my headphones on, so no one disturbs me and no one is the wiser, but it's a fantastic feeling to be undisturbed by the constant buzzing and pinging from Slack and emails.

—Kim H.

For me, my morning routine is the ultimate act of self-care. I make myself what I consider to be the best cup of coffee in NYC, then proceed to do my skin-care routine, and play dress-up until I'm ready for the day. As someone who always struggled with accepting her body, taking that extra time in the morning to show myself some love really makes all the difference.

—Alexander M.

It's so, so easy to keep saying yes to things, but I've found it's so, so essential to take some time for yourself, whatever that means to you. For me, that means taking one evening once a week all to myself. It doesn't matter what I do: sometimes that's going home and watching TV, sometimes that's taking a long walk, and sometimes that's cooking something good for me. This might sound lame, but I actually mark this time on my calendar. As my friend Greta told me once, "Plans with yourself are still plans."

—Kate W.

Meditating, showering, painting my nails, ripping off the bandage and taking care of my to-do list, intentional tea drinking, calling my mom, writing lists when I need to organize myself, taking time to worry/journal, singing out loud, and dancing . . . all these things help me recognize that I am a human, and among my goals, I have a basic need to feel good about my everyday experience.

—Shannon O.

I love to go on a long run first thing in the morning. Every day, I look forward to blasting my favorite music, taking the time to focus on my mind/body connection, and sweating out any negativity! I feel so accomplished afterward and my energy is always in the best place to tackle the day ahead.

—Penda N.

I watch *This Is Us* and *Grey's Anatomy* while ugly crying and giving myself a manicure. Very therapeutic. Best to do alone.

—Yon L.

I always make sure to wake up early enough to give myself 15 minutes to sit in silence before I head off to work. I wouldn't call it meditation, but more of a daily reflection. Doing so helps me put things into perspective and focus on what's important, and it's a needed respite before talking to people in an office for 9 ½ hours.

—Morgan R.

When I take a few minutes at the beginning of my day to plan out my tasks during the week, it helps me really focus on what's important. I can rule out things that are just minutiae and be more present when it matters. And if I have some downtime and am feeling creative, creating weekly or monthly spreads in my bullet journal helps me de-stress and unwind.

—Kathleen A.

ShiShi Rose

on reclaiming her body after loss

It seems the act of getting pregnant and staying pregnant is governed by luck. There's no real rhyme or reason to why some people cannot sustain pregnancies and others seem to do so flawlessly. Or rather, what seems flawless to outsiders. Some people have multiple unexplained losses, then go on to have numerous healthy children. None of it really makes sense. And all the prenatal vitamins, healthy eating, de-stressing, deep breathing, and teams of medical professionals cannot a healthy pregnancy guarantee.

No matter the reason for the loss, most of us with birthing bodies blame ourselves when things don't go well. I've lost two pregnancies in my life, and both times I heard this little voice in my head telling me I could have done something differently, or better. And if I had, maybe I would have a healthy baby in my arms. I labeled this loss as a failure on my part because that felt like the easiest thing to do. (Who else could I blame?) And then, subsequently, it felt easier to punish myself too. To treat myself as if I were undeserving of care or love or even trying again for another baby.

It wasn't until a few years ago that I started to learn more about the way my body works. It started a year after that last miscarriage. After what felt like a lifetime of abnormal periods, I started to wonder if the problem was deeper than just my physical being, if it was mental and spiritual too. That maybe how I viewed and treated my body was only worsening how it functioned.

Eventually it felt like I was doing a disservice to myself and the two almost-babies that had been growing in my womb to continue to live with the blame. During the past year and a half, I have dedicated my life to trauma work and healing. I went to a trauma treatment center for 2 months, and I learned how to speak about all the things that have happened. My therapist told me to kick and scream—so I did. I purged pain out. The process felt so impossible, but after leaving that space, I felt like I was doing the opposite of digging the grave I felt I had been sinking into. Rather, this time, I was crawling back into the world. This honoring of my body that started to unfold was something I'd needed for decades. Something that spanned so far past a first period or losses. And it wasn't just how I felt about my body, but my whole self. I'm not separate from her.

Because the healing process can be so painful, I realized I needed more things to calm my spirit. A safe landing space just for me. In private, I started dancing again. Dancing was something that got me through some of my hardest moments as a child; now it's what connects me to that little girl and brings me peace. I feel like I am home when I dance—I have found a home in my body and it's not a stranger anymore.

ShiShi is an activist, writer, and postpartum doula. Her work as an activist centers on racism, Black women's rights, and the elevation of the Black community by advocating for reparations and the consistent support of the Black family at birth and beyond.

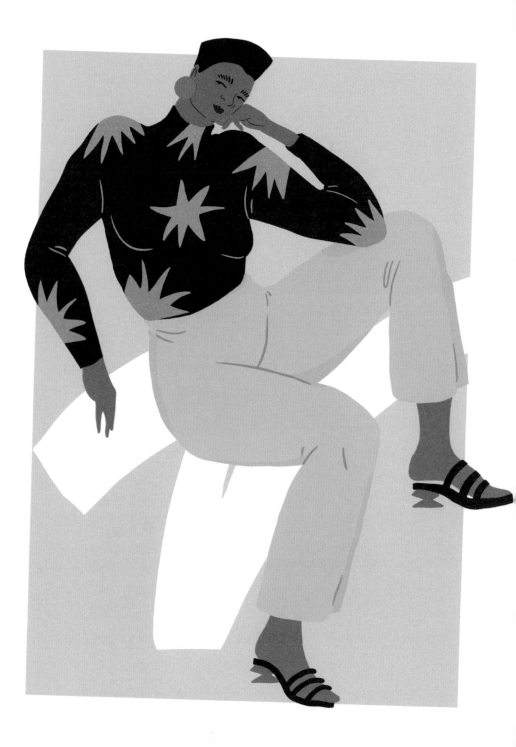

finding the right therapist for you

For many of us, therapy is an important part of maintaining our overall physical and mental wellness. Finding a therapist—especially one you like, who works for your needs—can be like searching for the perfect shade of red lipstick. No two are the same, and what works for your BFF might not work for you. But seriously, everyone benefits from finding the right one. It'll definitely take some work on your part, but taking care of you is always worth it. We put together some tips to get you started.

narrow your search

The only person who can decide what your mental health needs are is you. You can and should discuss your mental health with your primary care provider, and if they recommend an alternate course of action besides therapy (like medication), you should give that thoughtful consideration. With that being said, sit down and, as honestly as possible, think about (and write down) what you would like to work on. Social anxiety? Navigating a close relationship after sexual trauma? Struggling to connect to your partner? Ask your primary doctor or use resources like the American Psychiatric Association (APA) to help you research. You can also use sites like Zocdoc and Psychology Today to find therapists with those specialties in your area. You can ask your friends, and even if you don't see the same exact therapist as your friend (this could feel weird, especially if you're close), maybe someone else in their office will work for you.

Make a short list of your options based on who you think would be the best fit, and then start considering factors like schedule, location, and of course, price. You might find a therapist who feels like the perfect match but one of these issues becomes a deal breaker. If that happens, you can also try asking for a referral in their network.

figure out your finances

Worrying about money is probably the last thing you want to do when it comes to supporting your mental and emotional health—so get it out of the way as soon as possible.

First, check with your HR department and/or insurance provider to see whether mental health services are covered and under which conditions. After you've made your list of prospective therapists, call each office to see who will accept your insurance—this might make your choice a bit easier. If your insurance won't cover therapy outright, you can use an FSA, HSA, or HRA to help pay, or at least write off some of the cost on your taxes.

Once you know whether insurance will cover any part of therapy, figure out how much you can actually budget for therapy. Knowing what's doable moneywise will help you in the long run. No one wants to stop kick-ass therapy because of financial difficulties.

You should also think about how long you intend to be in therapy. Ideally, this won't be dictated by finances, but unfortunately, it might be. If you find that you can budget for a certain number of sessions with a therapist who is too expensive for long-term support, you can communicate your needs and what you would like to achieve in that limited time. Some therapists might also give a discount for "bundled" sessions.

A more affordable option worth exploring is online therapy. Remember, it's extremely important to do your research and make sure you're only giving your money to licensed professionals (definitely important IRL, too!).

start the conversation

There should be no need to jump right into a bunch of sessions—and it could be a red flag if an office is pressuring you to commit to appointments. Put together some questions with your personal needs in mind, then request an informal phone call or first meeting with your prospective therapist. I know, you'd probably rather just send an email, but try your best to do a call or face-to-face meeting—it'll be way easier to tell if you're vibing together. Don't forget to be forthcoming with them about your needs and goals, and be clear about any time or financial limitations.

be honest with yourself

A lot of people, especially women, feel pressure to stay in situations that make them uncomfortable—dates, conversations, interactions with weird strangers, and yup, unhelpful therapy. If you find you're feeling unproductively judged or unhappy, after you feel you've made an honest effort to be introspective, move on—whether it's the first or fifth or fifteenth time you've met with that therapist. You're not obligated to continue seeing someone if you genuinely feel they're not helping you or even if you're not feeling a connection with them. Your relationship with your therapist is a personal relationship like any other. Sometimes people just don't click, and that's OK!

Now that you've done the preliminary work, your next search will be less intimidating. Call the next name on your list. If necessary, contact your doctor and let them know it didn't work out, ask for help elsewhere in your network, or look up some new names on your own. When it's time to meet with the next therapist, don't be discouraged by poor previous experiences. Ask the same questions, and stick to your guns. You shouldn't be settling when it comes to your physical or mental healthcare—it's your time and money, after all. Practice patience, don't be discouraged, and be proud of yourself for taking your well-being into your own hands.

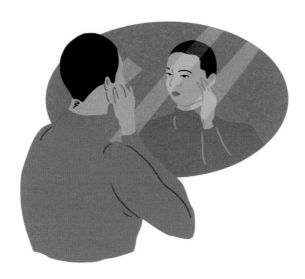

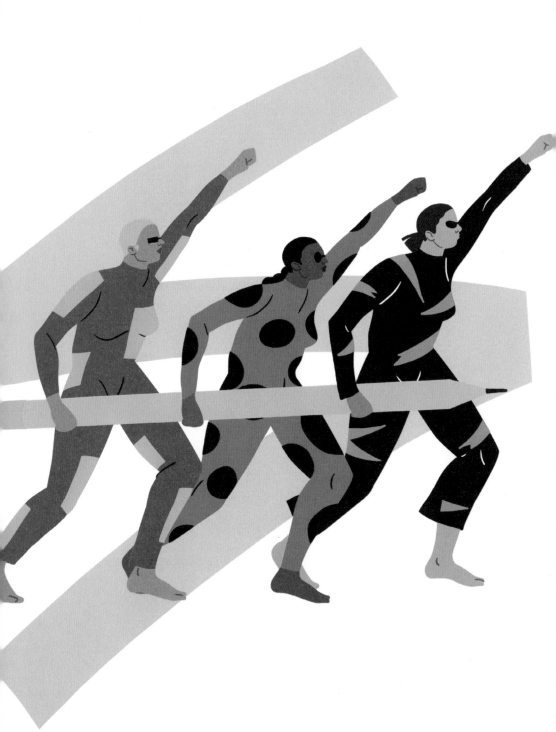

a patriarchy-proof reading list

As the ancient proverb goes, "Books rule, boys drool." Just kidding, unfortunately. Also unfortunately, the patriarchy is very real and very committed to maintaining a certain power structure in our culture (and all cultures, tbh). Functioning in a world with so much systemic oppression can be, to put it extremely mildly, pretty draining, which is why it's so important to find inspiration from others committed to dismantling the patriarchy and empowering people who are doing the same. We've still got work to do, so we put together a book list for the moments when we need a pick-me-up (or a rally cry) to keep fighting the good fight.

Are You My Mother? A Comic Drama **(2013) by Alison Bechdel.**
I read *Are You My Mother?* fresh out of college and just starting a new career as a fifth-grade special education teacher in the Bronx. Alison Bechdel's richly layered narrative gave me a much-needed introspective escape on my long, early morning commutes to a job rife with emotional labor. A meditation on her relationship with her mother, Bechdel's graphic novel weaves together memories, psychological theory, found letters, conversations, and other life ephemera to answer the question that tugs at us all: "How much of me is me?" And with appearances from writers (Virginia Woolf and P. D. Eastman), psychologists (D. W. Winnicott and Alice Miller), and her own work (*Dykes to Watch Out For*), Bechdel provides us, too, with a profound road map for unpacking identity and experience.

—Laura B.

Girl Sex 101 **(2015) by Allison Moon.** Scissoring, cunnilingus, strap-ons, lots of veiny dildos: These may or may not be positions/props used to depict lesbian sex in porn, your imagination, and the horny grapevine. I'm not here to shame anyone's kink (I def have some hardware of my own in a drawer at home); instead I will recommend a book that really opened my eyes to how we can demystify our idea of what having girl sex is. *Girl Sex 101* helped me improve my own communication, pleasure, and self-confidence with my lady lover. Out of any sex ed book I've ever read, this one takes the cake! The to-the-point illustrations help navigate female sexuality, and it features a working "road map" to facilitate your partner's pleasure. The entire book is consent focused and makes intimidating sex stuff more approachable! Not to mention, there are a lot of pro tips for the (not-to-be-forgotten) stereotypes above.

—Dani B.

Orlando: A Biography (1928) by **Virginia Woolf.** Virginia Woolf doesn't have a reputation for being a super sunny writer, so if you haven't read *Orlando*, you might be surprised to hear that it's actually soooo much fun! In a nutshell, it's basically an elaborate fan fiction Woolf wrote about her gal pal Vita Sackville-West and her family's history. The titular character, Orlando, is a gender nonconforming poet who lives for centuries and hangs out with a bunch of key figures from England's literary canon (while also casually switching out her gender and sex as time goes on). It's also a well-adapted movie starring Tilda Swinton, who was maybe put on this earth to play wonderful, androgynous characters like Orlando. (But of course, please read the book first!)

—Toni B.

Like A Mother: A Feminist Journey Through the Science and Culture of Pregnancy (2018) by **Angela Garbes.** Reading this book, I found myself yelling, "Yes! This girl gets it!" like every other page. Garbes shows mothers everywhere that it's OK to love the at-home, messy, chaotic, and tender moments of motherhood, but also mourn the evolution of your former pre-child self.

—Dr. Jenn

Stone Butch Blues (1993) by **Leslie Feinberg.** This is one of those books you'll feel emotional about every time it's mentioned after you're finished reading. *Stone Butch Blues* tells the extremely raw, heartbreaking, and tender story of Jess Goldberg, a butch human navigating gender (and violence) in small-town America before the Stonewall Riots. It's a book that's hard to put down once you've started—and it'll make you think a lot about oppression, authenticity, identity, growth, and kindness (y'know, a really light read!). Leslie Feinberg was an incredible storyteller and activist, and we're so lucky to have this work live on. It can be tough to find copies because it's out of print now, but the manuscript was available on Leslie's website for a long time as a free, downloadable PDF. No matter how you get your hands on the story, the effort is worth it, I promise.

—Brianna F.

additional reading

Ask Me About My Uterus: A Quest to Make Doctors Believe in Women's Pain (2018) by Abby Norman

Bad Feminist (2014) by Roxane Gay

Mama Glow: A Hip Guide to Your Fabulous Abundant Pregnancy (2012) by Latham Thomas

Modern HERstory: Stories of Women and Nonbinary People Rewriting History (2018) by Blair Imani

Nobody's Victim: Fighting Psychos, Stalkers, Pervs, and Trolls (2019) by Carrie Goldberg

Period Power: A Manifesto for the Menstrual Movement (2018) by Nadya Okamoto

Periods Gone Public: Taking a Stand on Menstrual Equity (2017) by Jennifer Weiss-Wolf

Pleasure Activism: The Politics of Feeling Good (2019) by adrienne maree brown

Shout Your Abortion (2018) by Amelia Bonow and Emily Nokes

The Vagina Bible: The Vulva and the Vagina: Separating the Myth from the Medicine (2019) by Jennifer Gunter

The Wonder Down Under: The Insider's Guide to the Anatomy, Biology, and Reality of the Vagina (2018) by Nina Brochmann and Ellen Støkken Dahl

online resources

Bedsider
bedsider.org

The Body Is Not an Apology
thebodyisnotanapology.com

The Labia Library
labialibrary.org.au

Planned Parenthood's educational resources
plannedparenthood.org/learn

Queering Reproductive Justice: A Toolkit
thetaskforce.org/wp-content/uploads/2017/03/Queering-Reproductive-Justice-A-Toolkit-FINAL.pdf

The Thinx Periodical
shethinx.com/pages/thinx-periodical

organizations
that deserve support

Advancing New Standards in Reproductive Health (ANSIRH)

An Oakland-based collaborative research group that conducts innovative, rigorous, multidisciplinary research on complex issues related to people's sexual and reproductive lives.

Center for Reproductive Rights

A global legal advocacy organization that seeks to advance reproductive rights.

Girls Inc.

A US nonprofit that inspires all girls to be strong, smart, and bold through direct service and advocacy, including mentoring relationships and research-based programming.

GiveRise

The Thinx Inc. give-back program that fights for better access to puberty education, amplifies grassroots activism around causes like menstrual equity, and donates to mission-aligned causes.

NARAL

A nonprofit organization that engages in political action and advocacy efforts to oppose restrictions on abortion and expand access to abortion.

PERIOD

The largest youth-run nonprofit fighting to end period poverty and period stigma through service, education, and advocacy.

Planned Parenthood

A nonprofit organization that provides comprehensive reproductive and sexual healthcare in the United States and globally.

Power to Decide

An organization that works to empower all young people with the resources they need to decide if, when, and under what circumstances to get pregnant and have a child.

The PRIDE Study

The first long-term national health study of LGBTQ+ people.

TIME'S UP Legal Defense Fund

Part of the TIME'S UP movement against sexual harassment, the fund provides legal defense for sexual violence victims, especially those who experience(d) misconduct in the workplace.

The Yellowhammer Fund

A member of the National Network of Abortion Funds, it provides funding for anyone seeking care at one of Alabama's three abortion clinics, assisting with other barriers to access, such as travel and lodging.

acknowledgments

A couple shout-outs to the village that
made this book happen:

First and foremost, Dr. Jenn Conti for sharing her words
and medical expertise. We could not have asked for a better
partner on this project. We bow down to our illustrator,
Daiana Ruiz. Many thanks to Samantha Panepinto for her
meticulously researched editorial contributions and our
kicka$$ editorial assistant, Penda N'diaye, for keeping us
organized and sane. Our deepest gratitude to our fearless
leaders Maria Molland and Siobhán Lonergan, who set the
bar for busting taboos every damn day. *The Vagina Book*
literally would not exist without Maeve Roughton kicking off
this project. The wonderful team at Chronicle: our fantastic
editor Rachel Hiles, our designer Vanessa Dina, and our
marketing and publicity team, Cynthia Shannon and Joyce
Lin. We'd also like to thank Jacob Molland for his legal advice,
and endless patience with answering emails.

<3 The Thinx Inc. Team

Words: Toni Brannagan, Hilary Fischer-Groban,
Brianna Flaherty

Design: Janet Chan, Meng Shui

PR: CJ Frogozo, Leesa Raab